THE HEALING POWER OF
SLEEP

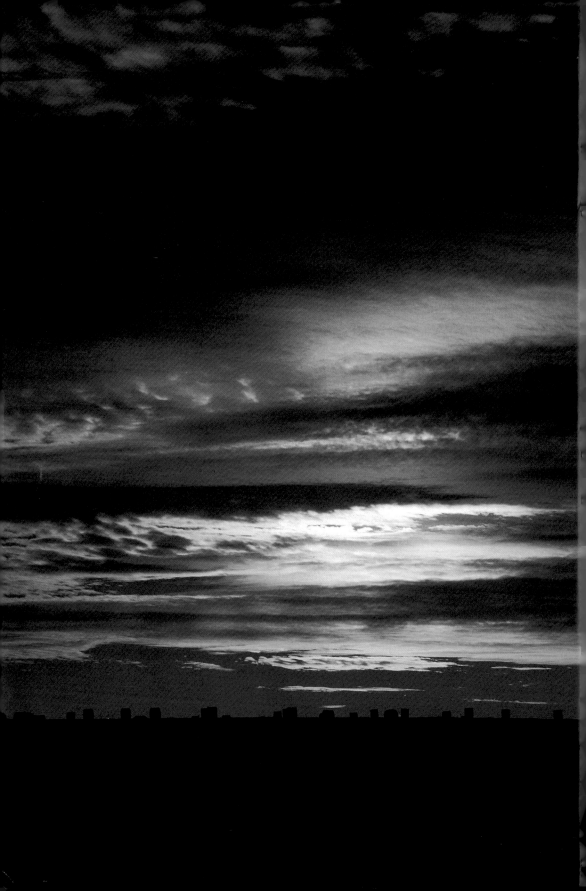

THE HEALING POWER OF
SLEEP

HOW TO ACHIEVE RESTORATIVE SLEEP NATURALLY

SHEILA LAVERY

A GAIA ORIGINAL

F

A Fireside Book
Published by Simon & Schuster Inc.

FIRESIDE
Simon & Schuster Inc.
Rockefeller Center
1230 Avenue of the Americas
New York, New York 10020

Designed by Phil Gamble

Printed in Singapore

10 9 8 7 6 5 4 3 2 1

Consultant

Dr Ronald Chisholm
Clinical Assistant Professor of Medicine and
Associate Director of the Sleep Disorders Center,
Indiana University Medical School, USA.

This book is not intended to replace medical care
under the direct supervision of a qualified doctor.
Before embarking on any changes in your health
regime, consult your doctor.

Library of Congress Cataloging-in-Publication Data

Lavery, Sheila, 1963-
    The healing power of sleep: how to achieve restorative sleep naturally / Sheila Lavery.
    p.   cm.
    "A Gaia original."
    "A Fireside book."
    "First published in the United Kingdom in 1997 by Gaia Books"--T.p. verso.
    Includes bibliographical references and index.
    ISBN 0-684-83352-2
    1. Sleep. 2. Insomnia. I. Title.
RA786.L38 1997
154.6--dc20   96-38605
                                CIP

ISBN 0-684-83352-2

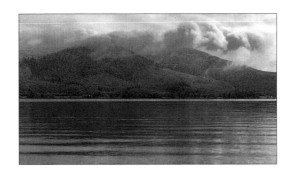

Contents

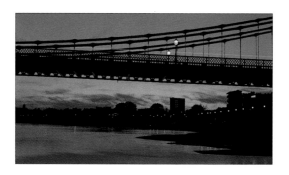

Foreword

Not poppy, nor mandragora,
Nor all the drowsy syrups of the world,
Shall ever medicine thee to that sweet sleep
Which thou ow'dst yesterday

William Shakespeare
1564-1616

Sheila Lavery has written a book that encompasses all of the aspects of sleep that fascinate us, including normal and abnormal sleep, changes with age, dreams, snoring, and much more. In addition to presenting the standard approaches, this work enlarges our grasp by covering alternative viewpoints including those provided by non-Western traditions. For example, yoga, herbs, flowers and aromatherapy are presented along with recently established behavioral and medication regimens for the treatment of insomnia. Of course the value of an approach is not equivalent to how exotic it may be, but this breadth of approach enables the reader to consider very

different strategies. Although the alternative approaches may not work for everyone, there is no question that different vantage points may offer new solutions for the vexations of sleeplessness. While the development of our understanding and practice of sleep hygiene, stimulus control, sleep restriction, cognitive and pharmacologic treatments have much to offer, the fact remains that insomnia continues to be one of the most common health complaints. Although the effectiveness of nutritional and herbal approaches to insomnia is not fully accepted by orthodox medicine, it is worthwhile to keep an open mind. For too many years Western scientists and medical practitioners neglected and minimized the importance of nutrition and vitamins for the prevention of heart disease and cancer. This book reminds us that sleep problems have been addressed for many years by many different cultures in many different ways, and we may benefit from this experience.

Insomnia is undertreated. In addition, the modern work ethos focuses on performance and productivity, stress pervades our daily lives, shift work is more common, and 24 hour access to media and the internet have resulted in a fatigued society. The insufficient or troubled sleeper may be pessimistic that anything can be done and so only one in twenty seeks help. Alternatively, the insomniac may assume that sleeping drugs are the only (and an unacceptable) answer and this precludes their receiving help. Even if an individual seeks help from a physician or psychologist the expertise thoroughly to evaluate, devise a comprehensive treatment plan, and spend sufficient time in systematic follow-up is an ideal that is rarely fulfilled. The field is attempting to address these problems by establishing a coherent body of knowledge, training health care practitioners in clinical sleep disorders, and promoting research. As these developments bear fruit individuals with sleep disturbance will no longer be on their own.

The Healing Power of Sleep will inform the general reader, not just those with sleep disorders, of the need to understand the fundamental role that good sleep practices play in the regulation of alertness, mood, mental processes, and performance. By addressing these pervasive problems, this book offers hope for a better quality of life.

Arthur J. Spielman, PhD
Director, Sleep Disorders Center
The City College of the City University of New York

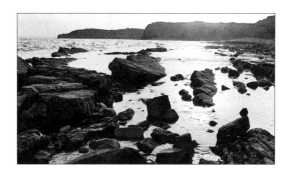

Introduction

"...dreams are a part of nature, which harbours no intention to deceive but expresses something as best it can, just as a plant grows or an animal seeks its food..."

Carl J. Jung
(1875-1961)

Sleep has been defined as "a natural state of relative unconsciousness and immobility recurring in man and animals at least once a day." The brevity of the definition reflects what little thought most of us give to this activity that occupies around a third of our lives and has a profound effect on our mental, emotional, and physical health. We think of sleep as little more than a period of rest that punctuates the activity of our lives. We mark the end of the day by going to bed, switching off to its problems and pleasures and, if we sleep well, we wake up refreshed and ready to get on with our conscious existence. Only when we sleep badly or dream vividly do we give a second thought to what happened during the night.

The philosopher Bertrand Russell is credited with saying that, "Men who are unhappy, like men who sleep badly are always proud of the fact." It is true that people who do not sleep well will always tell you so, but it may be because they find it unnatural, frustrating, and stressful, rather than a source of pride. Sleeping well may be something we take for granted, but sleeping badly can become an obsession. The number of sleep disorders associations, publications, and self-help groups around the world are testament to the fact that lack of sleep is a serious issue. Thanks to the work of psychiatrists, psychologists, and physiologists in sleep research laboratories we know something about what happens during sleep, but despite extensive research into the phenomenon we still have no clear cut answers to the most basic questions such as why we need to sleep and how important it really is to our health and happiness.

It does not take a research scientist to tell you that a night of disturbed sleep is distressing and that several disrupted nights can leave you feeling wretched. But we do rely on research to prove that sleep is fundamental to a healthy immune system, sound mental health, and the growth and repair of every cell in the body.

Science and nature are both great teachers, and the advice in this book is derived from both sources. It draws on the work of sleep specialists and "natural" therapists who understand that sleep problems most often arise from the way we live our lives, and should be treated as such. The aim of the book is to investigate sleep problems and their causes to enable you to recognize the factors that may lie at the heart of particular sleep problem. It also contains suggestions for changes you can make to your lifestyle to improve your quality of sleep and your health.

Every one of us has individual sleep needs and is affected by specific factors that influence our ability to sleep. The questionnaires on the following pages are intended as a starting point for discovering the nature of your particular problem, or indeed if you have a problem in the first place. By answering the questions honestly, you should be able to determine your sleep needs and pinpoint the principal factors that may be interfering with your sleep.

Subsequent chapters examine the sleep process and its function, and suggest numerous ways in which you can help yourself to achieve better sleep, naturally. Remember, better sleep is within everybody's grasp; it needs no magic pills or potions, just a little time and effort. Persevere in your quest for sound, restorative sleep, the investment is small when you consider the potential rewards in terms of improved physical, emotional, and mental wellbeing.

Questionnaire

Analysing your sleep problem

These short questionnaires are designed to help you to determine whether you have a sleep problem and, if so, what the probable causes are. In the unlikely event that you have worked through the questionnaires and found nothing that contributes to your particular problem, it is worth asking yourself if you really have a sleep problem or simply have unrealistic expectations. You may be a light sleeper, a short sleeper or perhaps you go to bed too early. It might help to keep a diary of what time you go to bed, what time you get up and how much time you spend asleep. A sleep diary kept over two or three weeks can often provide valuable insights.

1 DO YOU HAVE A SLEEP PROBLEM?

	Yes	No
Do you find it difficult to get to sleep?	A	B
Do you often wake during the night?	A	B
If you wake do you have difficulty getting back to sleep?	A	B
Do you wake up early in the morning, unable to get back to sleep?	A	B
Do you wake feeling unrefreshed?	C	D
Do you feel tired or drowsy during the day?	C	D
Do you feel dissatisfied with the amount of sleep you get?	C	D

One or more Cs

You appear to have a sleep problem that is affecting your health and happiness, and possibly your performance at work. Use Questionnaire 2 to find out if disturbed rhythms are at the root of your problem.

One or more As, three Ds

You appear to have some irregular sleep patterns, although these no not appear to be having a bad effect on your health at present. Questionnaire 2 may help you discover the cause of your irregular sleep habits.

Four Bs, three Ds

You appear to sleep well. Even if your sleep is occasionally disturbed, it does not seem to interfere with your mental or physical health or your ability to function during the day. If you continue to work well and feel good there is no need to worry about the occasional disturbed night.

2 IS YOUR SLEEP PROBLEM CAUSED BY DISTURBED RHYTHMS?

Do you go to sleep when you are not tired?	Yes/No
Do you often sleep late to catch up on lost sleep?	Yes/No
Do you go to bed at irregular times?	Yes/No
Do you work night shifts?	Yes/No
Do you take naps during the day?	Yes/No
Do you sleep in late at weekends ?	Yes/No
Are you looking after a young baby who wakes during the night?	Yes/No
Do you travel across time zones more than once a month?	Yes/No

One or more YES anwers

A lack of routine is likely to be the major cause of fatigue and unrefreshing sleep. Regular sleep habits form the basis of healing sleep. For more information on the importance of routine and compensating for lack of it, *see* Chapter Five.

All NO answers

Your sleep problem is unlikely to be attributable to disturbed rhythms. You seem to have a regular sleep routine so the cause of your problem lies elsewhere. It may be your health or lifestyle that is to blame. Try Questionnaire 3 to find out.

3 ARE HEALTH PROBLEMS AFFECTING YOUR SLEEP?

Are you overweight ?	Yes/No
Do you drink heavily – more than 28 (men) or 21 (women) small drinks a week?	Yes/No
Do you feel pain during the night?	Yes/No
Do you have a chronic or debilitating illness?	Yes/No
Do you ever wake during the night gasping for breath?	Yes/No
Are you taking any medications?	Yes/No
Have you been told that you snore loudly?	Yes/No

One or more YES answers

It is likely that health problems are contributing to your sleep disturbance. Discuss your sleep problem and any other health issues with your doctor.

All NO answers

Your physical health seems to be good and is not an obvious cause of your sleep problems. Your lifestyle and/or emotional health are more likely to be disturbing your sleep. *See* Questionnaire 4.

4 IS YOUR DAY SLEEP-FRIENDLY?

Do you take regular exercise?	Yes/No
Do you drink less than three cups of coffee a day?	Yes/No
Do you drink less than two small alcoholic drinks a day?	Yes/No
Do you avoid heavy meals late at night?	Yes/No
Are you a non-smoker?	Yes/No
Do you stop worrying about work when you get home?	Yes/No
Do you allow time to unwind before you go to bed?	Yes/No

One or more NO answers

It is likely that your daily routine is contributing to your sleep problem. You need to make some changes, but do not attempt to make too many changes at once. *See* Chapters Five and Eight for further information.

All YES answers

If you have a sleep problem, it is unlikely to be caused by your lifestyle. If your health is good and your sleep routine is sound, the problem may be an emotional one. *See* Questionnaire 5.

5 IS EMOTIONAL STRESS A FACTOR?

Do you feel unable to cope at work?	Yes/No
Do you have financial worries?	Yes/No
Do you have a problem with your main relationship?	Yes/No
Have you had a recent bereavement?	Yes/No
Is there illness in the family?	Yes/No
Are you worried about your children?	Yes/No
Do you feel depressed and worthless?	Yes/No
Do you feel constantly on edge?	Yes/No

One or more YES answers

It is likely that emotional stress is keeping you awake at night. Grief, depression, and anxiety are major causes of sleep disturbance. *See* Chapters Five and Six for further information and advice.

All NO answers

If you answered no to all of the above then you are unlikely to have a serious chronic sleep problem. If you feel that your sleep is not quite as good as you would like it to be, it may be that you sleep environment is not conducive to restful sleep. *See* Questionnaire 6.

6 IS YOUR BEDROOM CONDUCIVE TO SLEEP?

Is your bedroom separate from your living/working area?	Yes/No
Is your bedroom quiet?	Yes/No
Is your bedroom warm but not stuffy?	Yes/No
Is your bed comfortable?	Yes/No
Is your bedroom still dark in the mornings?	Yes/No
Have you banned television from your bedroom?	Yes/No
Do you feel good in your bedroom?	Yes/No
Does the colour of your room relax you?	Yes/No

No more than one NO answer

Your bedroom is probably conducive to sleep, although any "no" answer indicates room for improvement. Disturbed sleep may be due to another aspect of your health or lifestyle.

Two or more NO answers

You need to make some changes to your sleep environment. Chapter Nine should be your starting point in finding out what is wrong with your bedroom and how you can change it.

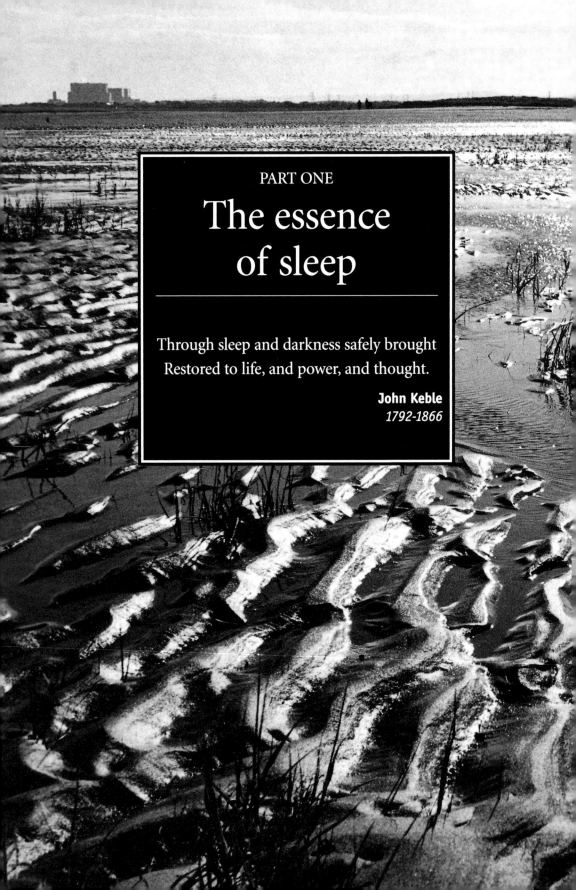

PART ONE

The essence
of sleep

Through sleep and darkness safely brought
Restored to life, and power, and thought.

John Keble
1792-1866

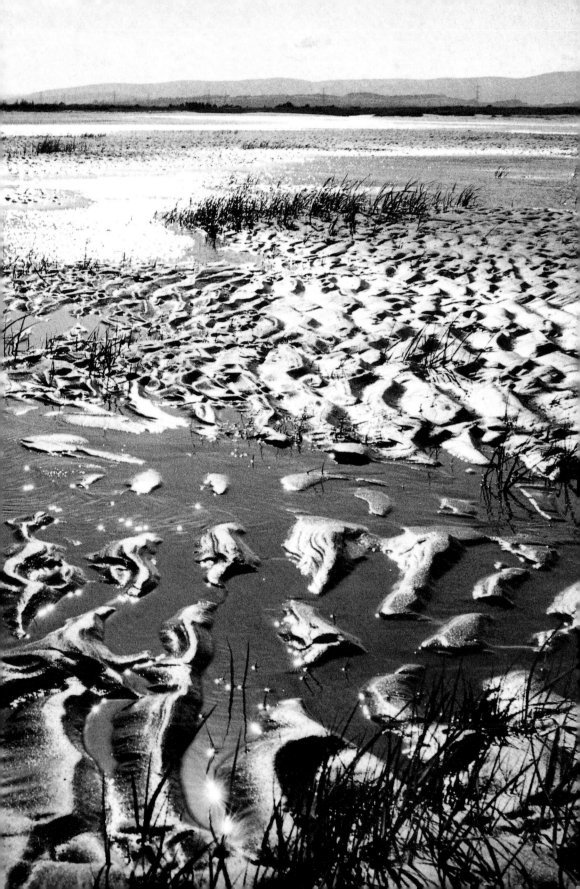

Chapter One

The restoration of wholeness

"Blessings on him who invented sleep, the mantle that covers all human thoughts, the food that satisfies hunger, the drink that slakes thirst, the fire that warms cold, the cold that moderates heat, and, lastly, the common currency that buys all things, the balance and weight that equalizes the shepherd and the king, the simpleton and the sage."

Miguel de Cervantes
(1547-1616)

Sleeping is as natural and essential as eating. Most people sleep for at least a short time in a 24-hour period, and the person who never sleeps has yet to be born. Although nobody is completely sure how sleep benefits our health, it is accepted that it does. There is also evidence that the converse is true: that lack of sleep makes us function less well. A mass of physiological and psychological evidence suggests a variety of possible mechanisms through which sleep maintains wellbeing. Laboratory experiments over the past 100 years show that animals such as rats and dogs die if they are denied sleep – the younger the animal the more vulnerable they are. But we have yet to find out if insomnia can be fatal in humans. What we do know is that even marginal lack of sleep can leave us feeling and functioning below par, and chronic lack of sleep can impair growth, reduce immunity to infection, and seriously affect our ability to concentrate and to make complex decisons.

At a basic level, sleep is a natural response to fatigue. The activity of the body slows down and the body and brain are able to rest. But sleep provides a qualitatively different kind of respite than that achieved when you rest without sleeping. Research over the past few decades has shown that a whole range of physical processes alter during sleep, and while the implications of some of these changes on health are easily understood, the purpose and effect of much of what happens to the body and brain during sleep still remains a mystery, open to scientific and philosophical speculation.

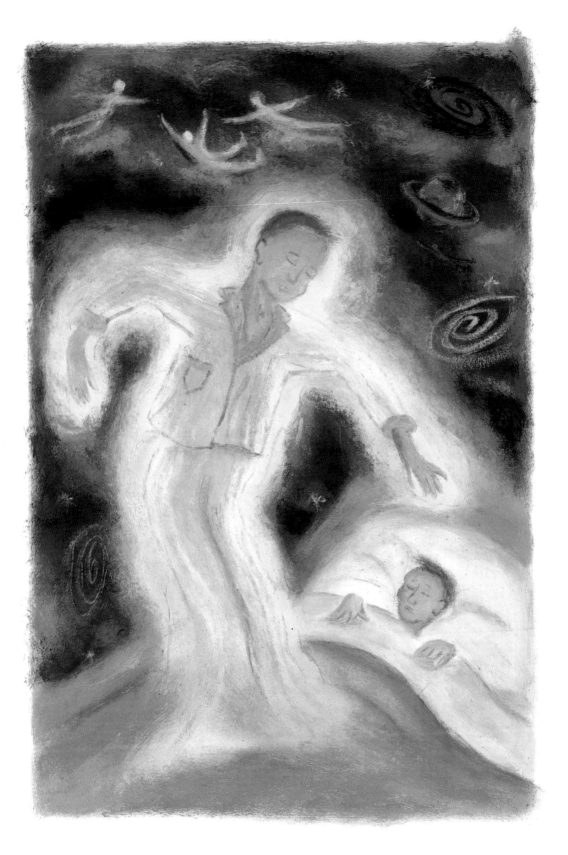

Restorative hormones

During wakefulness, the body burns oxygen and food to provide energy for the whole range of physical and mental activities. This "catabolic" state, in which more energy is spent than conserved, uses up body resources. The action of stimulating hormones – principally adrenaline (epinephrine) and natural corticosteroids – predominates. During sleep, we can be said to move into an "anabolic" state in which energy conservation, repair, and growth processes take over. Levels of adrenaline and corticosteroids – which counter anabolic activity – drop, and the body starts to produce growth hormone.

There is a great deal of evidence on the importance of sleep for growth and normal development in children. Reports showing that some abused children do not grow very well, have led some experts to suggest that this is because they are too afraid to sleep or wake too frequently to have sufficient deep sleep, during which growth hormone is released. When the same children start to sleep well in a more secure environment, their growth and development improve.

Growth hormone also serves an important purpose in adulthood, but instead of facilitating growth and development, it enables the body to renew and repair itself. Every tissue in the body from skin cells and blood cells to brain cells appears to be renewed faster during sleep than at any time while we are awake.

Promoting healing

Recent research seems to agree with the traditional belief that sleeping more during times of infectious illness helps us fight the infection and recover more quickly. Most people know what it is like to go to bed feeling ill and feverish and wake refreshed. Excessive sleepiness is a natural consequence of practically all infectious diseases. This may be due to the effect of the immune system's increased production of certain proteins in response to the infection.

Adequate sleep may also play a role in helping us
to resist infection. Studies of healthy young adults have
shown that even moderate amounts of sleep deprivation
can reduce the levels of white blood cells thereby reducing
the effectiveness of the body's defence systems.

Psychological benefits

Sleep is believed by some psychologists to be a time
when repressed emotional issues are dealt with. Through
dreams, they argue, we are able to throw out useless
mental clutter and deal with emotions such as anger
and frustration so that these emotions are not repressed
to the point where they can become damaging.
Psychosomatic illness (physical illness with a psychological
origin) is believed to account for many disorders such as
high blood pressure, headaches, and stomach ulcers.
Dealing with emotional issues through dreams may help
to prevent repressed emotions such as anger, grief, and
jealousy from manifesting as physical symptoms.

Sleep and ideas of energy

According to eastern medical traditions such as the
Chinese system of medicine and India's system of
Ayurvedic medicine, we are composed of energy and
designed to function in harmony with planetary and
universal energy. As such we are guided by the cycles of
nature and light and dark. And just as the rest of nature
rests and repairs itself at night, so do we.

The Chinese approach

In traditional Chinese philosophy we are seen as living
between heaven and earth. The energies of heaven and
earth mingle within us to provide the energy for life.
For good health, this balance of heaven and earth within
us must be kept in harmony. To illustrate the idea of
harmony, the Chinese use the metaphors of *yin* and *yang*
to describe how the energy (*qi*) that exists within everything in the universe, is divided into two opposing yet

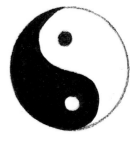

Yin and Yang
In traditional Chinese medicine
Yin represents female, dark, cool,
and solid characteristics. *Yang*
qualities are the reverse: male,
light, warm, and insubstantial.
Those with predominantly *yang*
characteristics tend to have little
sleep, whereas *yin* types are
lethargic and sleepy.

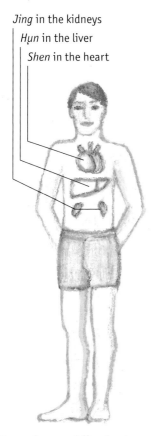

Jing in the kidneys
Hun in the liver
Shen in the heart

Hun, shen, and jing in sleep
Within the body, *hun* is stored in the liver and it returns there at night to allow peaceful sleep. During sleep, *shen* is supposed to reside in the heart and *jing* in the kidneys. This makes for harmony in body and mind, so sleep is peaceful, and growth and development take place.

complementary forces. We, and all of nature, are governed by these energetic forces.

Yin and *yang* energies also govern the three treasures of which the Chinese believe we are made: energy (*qi*), spirit (*shen*), and essence (*jing*). Energy is the force that moves, warms, and protects; without it life would cease. *Shen* is responsible for consciousness and mental abilities, and *jing* is responsible for growth, development, and reproduction. If there is an imbalance in the body as in the case of illness or stress, *shen* and *jing* have no residence during sleep, therefore growth and renewal cannot take place and the mind is not quiet.

The ethereal soul

Ancient Chinese ideas of sleep and dreams also include the concept of the wellbeing of the ethereal soul, known as *hun*. The Chinese believe that we have more than one soul, but the ethereal soul is the one that influences sleep and dreaming. *Hun* broadly corresponds to the Christian concept of soul or spirit, as it enters the body shortly after birth and when we die it flows back to heaven. Classic Chinese texts also suggest that *hun* follows the mind, so that if the mind is unconscious (as in the case of deep sleep), *hun* is "swept away". Modern Chinese thought, however, perceives *hun* as another level of consciousness, related to, but separate from the mind.

Thus the length and quality of sleep is related to *hun*. *Hun* is stored in the liver and it returns there at night. If there is an imbalance in the liver, it wanders, causing restless sleep and exhausting dreams.

During sleep *hun* is believed to collect images and ideas from the universal mind and present them to the mind of the individual as dreams. If sleep is sound and *hun* is flowing freely, images from the universal mind will keep you mentally and spiritually happy and creative. However, unsettled *hun* severs the link between the individual and universal minds and the individual loses creativity and becomes confused, isolated, and dreamless.

The Ayurvedic system

The traditional Indian medical system of Ayurveda is believed to be at least 5,000 years old. In Ayurveda the body is not seen as an isolated entity, but a vibrating bundle of energy with an innate intelligence that forms part of the continuous flow of energy that makes up nature. All things in nature, including ourselves, are composed of the three vital energies or *doshas*: *vata*, *pitta*, and *kapha*. Each *dosha* has its own qualities and although we are a mix of all three, everyone's physical and psychological constitution is based on one or two predominant *doshas*. The characteristics of each *dosha* are summarized in the panel right.

Nature works in cycles and rhythms and our bodies operate likewise. According to Ayurveda, sleeping well depends on staying in harmony with the fundamental energies of nature: balanced *doshas* produce perfect health and perfect sleep. But *doshas* can become imbalanced due to poor diet, stress, and numerous other factors, including not living in harmony with nature.

The doshas

Vata people are thin, excitable, tire easily, and have light, interrupted sleep. They tend to have irregular sleep habits and are prone to insomnia.

Pitta people are of medium build, get angry or irritable when stressed, tend to wake during the night feeling hot or thirsty, but usually wake up feeling alert.

Kapha people are solidly built, calm, affectionate, and slow moving. They love to sleep, their sleep tends to be heavy and prolonged and they wake up slowly.

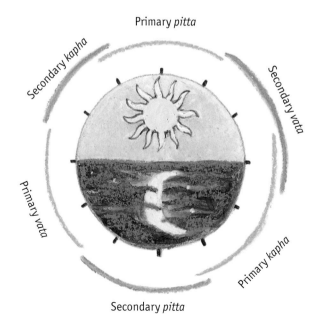

Primary *pitta*

Secondary *kapha*

Secondary *vata*

Primary *vata*

Primary *kapha*

Secondary *pitta*

The Ayurvedic clock

Throughout the day and night we go through primary and secondary periods of time when either *vata*, *pitta*, or *kaphā* energies predominate. Ayurveda advises that we try to go to sleep in *kapha* time (6pm – 10pm), when nature itself is slow and sleepy, and wake up in active and energetic *vata* time, which is before 6am.

The significance of dreams

Historical records are littered with references to the importance of sleep and dreams in ancient cultures. Many ancient cultures saw sleep either as a time when the soul left the body to commune with the spirits and the gods, or as a time when the body was visited by spirits, gods, or demons. Many early Christian thinkers believed that God revealed his will through dreams before Protestant reformers claimed their only virtue was in showing us our sins.

Yet dreams were not only valued for their religious significance. Many ancient societies considered dreams important for the maintenance of health and wellbeing. The ancient Greeks built shrines to Hypnos the god of sleep, and many of these were used as centres of healing. According to legend, the sick who visited the shrines were lulled to sleep by Hypnos and in their dreams they were visited by Asclepius, the god of medicine and healing. Asclepius offered advice, herbal remedies, and sometimes instant cures for the sick dreamer.

The Greek philosopher Plato believed that dreams could be of psychological significance. The father of medicine Hippocrates, the philosopher Aristotle, and the famous physician Galen all believed that dreams reflected the state of the body and could therefore be used to diagnose and treat illness.

The native Americans believed there was only a narrow division between the states of waking and dreaming, while the aboriginal peoples of Australia saw the universe as being made up of dreams. Both cultures believed in sharing and acting out dreams to release emotional and creative energy. Failure to do so created disharmony and a feeling of dissatisfaction with life. Indeed, dreams were considered vital to success in all areas of life, and it was through dreams that shamans (witchdoctors or medicine men) gained knowledge that would be used for the good of the tribe. Dreamers also called on a supernatural being known as a dream guide to take them through the dream world.

A common belief among traditional cultures was that sleep was a time when the soul or spirit broke free from the constraints of body, time, and space, enabling the dreamer to do, see, and feel life-enriching things that he or she would not experience in waking life. The suspension of conscious thought and physical activity that characterize sleep is frequently said to open the mind and body to energies from the universe, or divine revelations.

Belief in the spiritual significance of sleep and dreams has never really died out. Many of the ancient concepts have been translated into modern equivalents. In some branches of modern psychology, for example, the native American's dream guide would probably be seen as an unacknowledged aspect of the self, while dream sharing and enactment can be seen as forerunners of the concept of psychodrama.

Many people who believe their dreams are rich with emotional and spiritual meaning have turned to ancient traditions, in order to gain an understanding of how to work with dreams. Primitive cultures shared a common understanding that sleep and dreams play a very real and significant role in our health. By appreciating our need for a healthy quota of both, we can learn to enhance our mental, physical, and emotional wellbeing.

Dreams and spirituality
In this 16th-century Persian image, the sleeper is shown reaching spiritual fulfilment while dreaming.

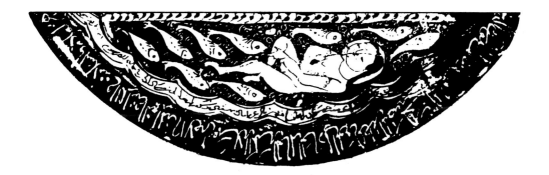

Chapter Two

Rhythms of sleep and waking

We live in a world that is constantly changing and evolving. But since the dawn of time, one natural phenomenon has remained completely predictable: that night must follow day. We know for certain that within a 24-hour cycle there will be a period of light and a period of dark.

People and animals also have an inbuilt body clock that governs a number of different physiological processes and which runs in parallel to external daily rhythms. In a primitive world this would have ensured that we remained awake and active during periods of light and warmth and rested in the cool of the night. With the advent of electric light, our periods of activity and rest are no longer determined exclusively by natural light and dark, but this biological clock, or biorhythm, ticks on. Even if you spend the evening in a brightly lit room, your internal clock seems to "know" that night is coming and prepares you for rest. Sleep researchers call this clock the circadian rhythm.

The circadian rhythm

The term circadian rhythm, comes from the Latin *circa diem*, meaning "about a day". As the name suggests, it works roughly on a 24-hour cycle. The circadian rhythm regulates all the rhythms of the body from the digestion and elimination processes, to the growth and renewal of cells, and to the rise and fall in body temperature. All these body rhythms are triggered by the action of a network of chemical messengers and nerves under the control of the circadian clock.

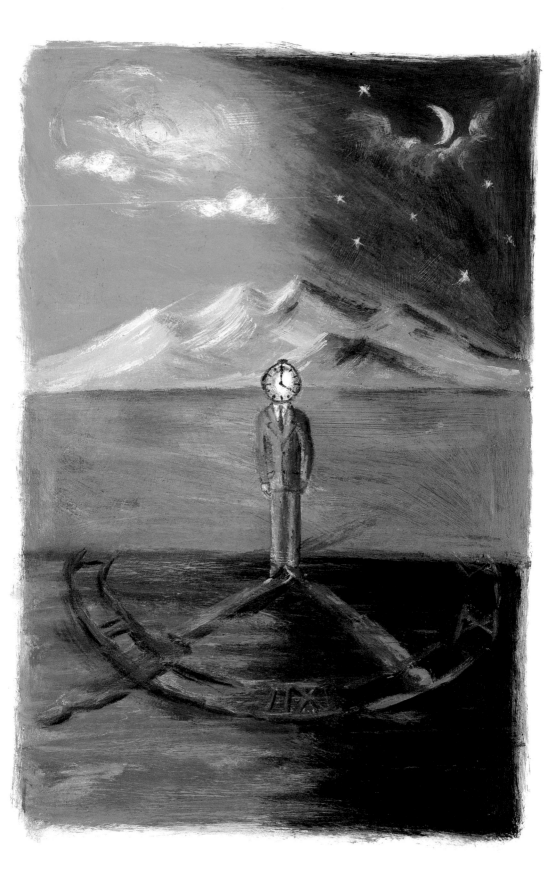

The clock itself is housed in a part of the brain called the suprachiasmatic nucleus. In complex creatures such as ourselves, this is located in the hypothalamus at the base of the brain, above the pituitary gland (*see* p.27). The pituitary gland is known as the master gland because it controls hormone production in the body.

In the 1940s scientists set out to prove that our sleep rhythms were governed by this internal clock and not simply by the effects of light and dark. Isolation studies conducted on animals and birds convinced them of it. Birds were exposed to continuous bright light for weeks, yet they maintained their normal patterns of sleep and wakefulness. Further studies on humans who elected to spend three to four weeks in an underground bunker produced similar results. The bunker was permanently illuminated, at times more brightly than others, but the volunteers maintained a regular routine of waking and sleeping within a cycle slightly longer than 24 hours.

Zeitgebers

The circadian rhythm ensures that body functions and sleep patterns run to a cycle of approximately 24 hours, irrespective of our environment. Some people are governed by a rhythm of slightly longer than 24 hours, for others it is slightly shorter. External factors, known as *zeitgebers* or "time-givers" keep us running to the same 24-hour cycle. Light and dark, activity and inactivity, noise and silence can all act as *zeitgebers*. Without such external stimuli, we would sleep and wake at regular intervals as dictated by our internal circadian rhythm, simply because that is how our bodies are programmed to work. However, *zeitgebers* regulate these rhythms so that we all go to sleep around the same time and get up at similar times. For example, if you were to stay awake all night, you could probably fall asleep at any given time during the next day. This would upset your biological time-keeping system and it could take a few days to right itself. However, forcing your body to override its natural

Infradian rhythms

Like animals that hibernate, humans are affected by the cycle of the seasons – a pattern know as the infradian rhythm. Our inbuilt tendency to get up when it is light and go to sleep when it is dark naturally lends itself to sleeping longer in winter and less in summer. Even those who no longer rely on natural light for the day's activities are affected by seasonal change, and sleep slightly longer in winter. This can be at least partly explained by the effect of dark winter evenings that make us feel that it is later than it really is and dark mornings that make us less inclined to wake up early.

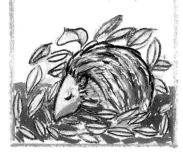

inclinations using *zeitgebers*, allows the previous rhythm quickly to re-establish itself. The easiest way to do this is to try to stay awake during the day and go to sleep at your normal time that night.

Body temperature and hormones

The graphs on p.26 show how body temperature and hormone levels fluctuate according to the circadian rhythm. During sleep the low levels of adrenaline and corticosteroids (*see* p.16) allow the body to make best use of the increased levels of growth hormone released by the pituitary gland at night. Its cell-renewing and protein

Overriding the body clock

You can force your body to override the body clock by the use of *zeitgebers* (*see* facing page). This is necessary, for example, when adjusting to a new time zone. Initially you are out of step with everyone else. You are tired at the wrong times. Your sleep needs, appetite, bowel activity, and body temperature are governed by your biological clock, which is not in keeping with the inhabitants of that time zone. After a few days the *zeitgebers* begin to ensure that your sleeping and waking times fit in with those of the people around you.

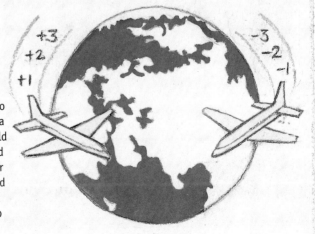

Jet lag is a familiar example of a confusion of the body clock. If you were to fly from London to New York you would add an extra five hours to your day: you would be tired early in the evening and wake early in the morning. After adjusting, your body clock would still run on a 24-hour cycle, but not the same 24 hours it kept to in London.

building effects are counteracted by the effects of adrenaline and corticosteroids. Ensuring regular periods of sleep at night allows the body clock to co-ordinate hormone production, so that the hormones work in harmony and we stay alert during the day and enjoy restorative sleep during the night. Most people go to sleep in the late evening when their corticosteroid levels are at their lowest and as body temperature and adrenaline levels start to drop. Going to bed at this time seems to increase the chances of a full night's sleep. Even when you are exhausted, it is more difficult to remain asleep after 5am because body temperature and the levels of stimulating hormones are on the increase.

Daily cycles

In the evening, body temperature and levels of adrenaline and corticosteroids, the hormones associated with wakefulness and activity, start to fall and we feel tired. Body temperature continues to fall throughout the night and drops to its lowest level – about 1°C (0.5°F) below its evening level – at 5am. It is tempting to think that our temperature drops because of the inactivity of lying in bed, but in fact it drops anyway. When you stay up all night your body temperature still remains lower than it is during the day, but not quite as low as it would be if you were asleep. The time of lowest body temperature (around 5am) is also the time at which you feel most tired, because it coincides with the time of lowest adrenaline.

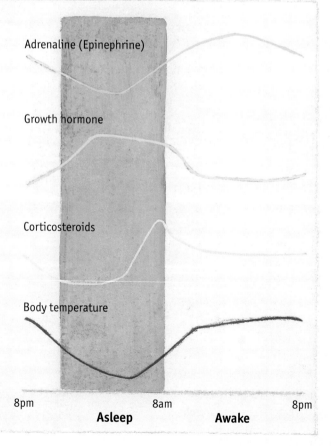

Adrenaline (Epinephrine)

Growth hormone

Corticosteroids

Body temperature

8pm

8am

8pm

Asleep

Awake

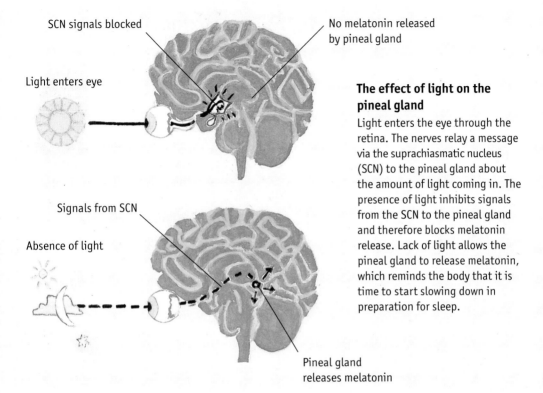

SCN signals blocked

No melatonin released by pineal gland

Light enters eye

Signals from SCN

Absence of light

Pineal gland releases melatonin

The effect of light on the pineal gland

Light enters the eye through the retina. The nerves relay a message via the suprachiasmatic nucleus (SCN) to the pineal gland about the amount of light coming in. The presence of light inhibits signals from the SCN to the pineal gland and therefore blocks melatonin release. Lack of light allows the pineal gland to release melatonin, which reminds the body that it is time to start slowing down in preparation for sleep.

The role of melatonin and the pineal gland

The ability of hibernating animals to sleep throughout the winter hinges on how their pineal gland responds to light. The pineal gland is a pea-sized gland deep in the brain that secretes a hormone called melatonin during darkness. The action of melatonin, which is sometimes called the sleep hormone, helps to control body rhythms and sleep-wake cycles.

The reduction in daylight hours, as winter approaches, triggers sufficient melatonin release in hibernating animals to enable them to sleep through the winter. In other animals and in humans, the daily fluctuation in melatonin levels helps to regulate the 24-hour cycle. Melatonin supplements may help to reset the internal body clock thereby inducing sleep when it is needed. This can be useful for helping shiftworkers, for example, to readjust their circadian rhythms (*see* p.22).

The stages of sleep

Before the introduction of brain-wave monitoring, our knowledge about the cycles of sleep was negligible. The development of electroencephalogram (EEG) machines to record electrical activity in the brain, and their use in sleep laboratories with other forms of monitoring, has enabled scientists to define different types, or stages, of sleep, and monitor the cycles of these different stages, linking the activity of the brain with other physiological changes at each stage.

We now know that all sleep is not the same. During our normal sleep cycle we snooze through periods of light sleep, drift into sleep so deep it is difficult to wake up, and spend some time in what is sometimes known as "dreaming sleep". There are several ways of categorizing the stages of sleep. Perhaps the most useful broad division is between rapid eye movement (REM) and non-REM (NREM) sleep. These two types of sleep alternate throughout the night under the guidance of the ultradian rhythm (*see* p.31). The table on the facing page summarizes the different physiological and mental features of the different stages of sleep

NREM sleep

NREM sleep, as implied by the alternative name orthodox sleep, is a time when body and brain behave exactly as you would expect during sleep: most of the muscles relax, body systems take a rest, and the brain waves associated with wakefulness and alertness (beta waves) disappear and are replaced by the increasingly slow, deep (delta) waves of inactivity.

NREM sleep accounts for an average of about 70 per cent of the total sleep time of a young adult. It is divided into four stages. Stages one and two are sometimes classed as light sleep, three and four as deep or slow-wave sleep.

In the first stage, which is really a state of semi consciousness, we feel drowsy and may experience a drifting or floating sensation. We may also have what are known

Sleep monitoring

Modern sleep monitoring systems record brain-wave activity by means of electroencephalogy (EEG) and take readings of eye movements with electroculographic (EOG) machinery, and muscle movements with electromyographic (EMG) machinery. EEG readings are taken by placing two electrodes on the scalp and recording the electrical activity of the brain. EOG readings are taken by taping electrodes above each eyebrow or on each cheekbone. EMG readings are taken from under the chin, where they record electrical activity in neck muscles.

Sleep stage characteristics

	NREM sleep *(stages one and two)* Light sleep	NREM sleep *(stages three and four)* Deep sleep	REM sleep
Physiological changes	♦ Slight muscle relaxation ♦ Eyes roll	♦ Growth hormone released ♦ Blood cells and body tissues rebuilt, especially skin ♦ Energy levels restored	♦ Irregular breathing and heart beat ♦ Increased blood flow and renewed protein levels in brain ♦ Blood pressure fluctuates ♦ Eyes move rapidly ♦ Face twitches ♦ Little body movement ♦ Increased testosterone release ♦ Women have increased blood flow to the vagina; men have erections
Changes in consciousness	♦ Preceded by drowsiness and less logical thinking ♦ Hypnogogic (dream-like) experiences ♦ Dreams remembered if woken	♦ Difficult to wake ♦ No conscious thought ♦ Some dreaming ♦ No memory of dreams or other events during sleep if woken	♦ Easily woken ♦ No conscious thought ♦ Most dreaming ♦ Dreams remembered if woken
Sleep disorders	♦ Most bedwetting and some sleep-talking in stage 2 ♦ Teeth-grinding	♦ Sleep-walking ♦ Sleep-talking ♦ Night terrors	♦ Nightmares ♦ Least sleep-talking
Special sleep requirements	♦ Short sleepers have very little of this sleep	♦ Short sleepers have near normal amounts of this sleep ♦ More needed during pregnancy, adolescence, after exercise or loss of sleep, in people with overactive thyroid gland ♦ Less is needed in those with underactive thyroid gland	♦ Short sleepers have near normal amounts of this sleep
Changes maintained throughout night	♦ Lowered body temperature ♦ Melatonin release ♦ Muscle relaxation ♦ Slow heart rate ♦ Low digestive and urinary activity ♦ Low adrenaline release ♦ Lowered blood pressure		

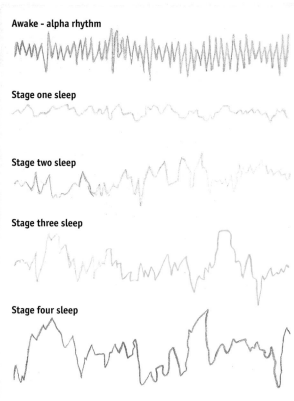

Awake - alpha rhythm

Stage one sleep

Stage two sleep

Stage three sleep

Stage four sleep

Types of brain wave

Awake When relaxed but awake, alpha rhythms as shown here predominate.
Stage one sleep brain activity is shown on EEGs as wavy lines of fairly regular small undulations which suggest mental relaxation.
Stage two sleep bursts of brain activity lasting only a second or two appear on the EEG. These "sleep spindles" are what characterize this stage. As stage two merges into stage three, the brain waves continue to deepen into mostly large, slow waves – the larger and slower the brain waves the deeper the sleep.
Stage three sleep between 20 and 50 per cent of brain waves are slow (delta) waves.
Stage four sleep is reached when over 50 per cent of the waves are slow.

as hypnogogic experiences – dream-like sensations of falling, hearing voices, or seeing flashes of pictures. At the beginning of the night, stage one sleep lasts for one to ten minutes, and accounts for only about five per cent of total sleep time.

Stage two is the first stage of true sleep and accounts for about 50 per cent of total sleep. A healthy young adult normally reaches stage three, the first stage of deep sleep, within 20 minutes of lying down to sleep and spends only about seven per cent of total sleep time in this stage. Stage four is the deepest level of sleep and the one in which the body is believed to carry out most of its repair and restoration work. Most adults spend about 11 per cent of sleep time in stage four.

REM sleep

REM sleep is usually thought of as being distinct from the other four stages. It was first identified in 1957 by American sleep experts Nathaniel Kleitman and William Dement and was given the name "paradoxical" sleep because the high level of brain activity and the rapid eye movements observed appeared in surprising contrast with the degree of muscle relaxation to the extent of virtual paralysis. It has been suggested that this paralysis is a clever device that lets the mind explore the realms of its subconscious, while preventing us from acting out dream events that may include acts of violence and murder, which we would never carry out while conscious. During REM sleep blood flow to the brain is increased. In children this may enable the brain to grow and in adults to repair itself.

Healthy young adults first experience REM sleep within about 90 minutes of falling asleep. It recurs about every 90 minutes throughout the night and each time it recurs we spend a little longer in the REM stage, finishing with about 30 minutes of REM sleep just before we wake.

Sleep cycles

Research has shown that we sleep in cycles of 90 to 100 minutes. When we go to sleep, we normally pass through stages one, two, three, and four and then go back to stage two before going into the first REM sleep of the night. The time up to the beginning of the first REM stage makes up the first sleep cycle.

The second cycle starts with the first period of REM and continues through the four stages of NREM sleep until the second REM stage begins. Each cycle, which runs from the beginning of one block of REM sleep to the beginning of the next, typically lasts for 90 minutes. Every cycle, except the first, contains both REM and NREM sleep. In the first half of the night there is more deep (stages three and four) sleep than REM sleep, in the second half of the night, there is more REM sleep.

Daytime "sleep" cycles

In 1963 eminent American sleep researcher Nathaniel Kleitman suggested that the 90-minute "ultradian" cycle of REM and NREM sleep continues throughout the day, and laboratory experiments have shown that this may well be the case. In practical terms this means that roughly every 90 minutes we have a dip in energy and concentration levels, and these are times when we could easily fall asleep. Some experts believe insomniacs have difficulty sleeping because they miss this window of sleepiness and have to wait for it to recur.

The first period of REM sleep is quite short – usually lasting less than 15 minutes. As the night progresses, the periods of REM become progressively longer. Finally, in the last sleep cycle, which for most people is the fifth cycle, there is a block of REM sleep that lasts about half an hour. Healthy people do not go straight into REM sleep after a period of wakefulness, even if they have been woken from REM sleep. It normally takes about 30 minutes for REM sleep to recur.

The 90-minute cycles of REM sleep, alternating with orthodox sleep are known as ultradian rhythms. This pattern of sleep is universal. Nobody has ever been known to take all of their deep sleep or REM sleep in one block. Moreover, while a disrupted or unhealthy waking life can affect the quantity and quality of your sleep, it does not disrupt this pattern.

Various views have been expressed on whether NREM sleep is more important than REM sleep or vice versa. Experiments in sleep laboratories during the 1960s showed that people deprived of REM sleep on successive nights seemed to have a greater need for this type of sleep when they went back to sleep, and became more tense, irritable and lacked concentration when deprived of it. At the time it was believed that dreaming only occurred during REM sleep, and that these experiments therefore showed that dream deprivation could lead to severe mental disturbance.

We now know that dreaming occurs to some extent at all stages of sleep and so it may not be lack of dreams, but deprivation of some other aspect of REM sleep that causes the mental disturbance. However, it remains clear that for some reason we need this type of sleep and when deprived of it we will

Night-time sleep cycles

During a typical night we pass through the different stages of sleep in roughly 90-minute cycles. Proportionately more deep (stage three and four) sleep occurs in the early part of the night, and periods of REM sleep are longer in the latter part.

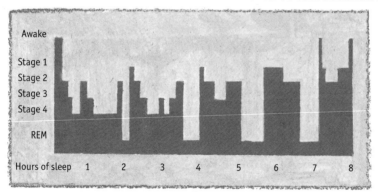

Awake
Stage 1
Stage 2
Stage 3
Stage 4
REM
Hours of sleep   1   2   3   4   5   6   7   8

always try to make up the loss the following night.

NREM sleep is also essential to health, in particular, stage four. In laboratory studies naturally short sleepers (people who remain well with less than five hours' sleep a night) were shown to have less stage one, two, and three sleep than average, but had average amounts of stage four and REM sleep.

It is now generally accepted that we need both NREM and REM sleep for good health. However, the precise physiological and mental role that each type of sleep fulfils is not yet fully understood. It is assumed that the high level of growth hormone released during NREM deep sleep is vital for physical health, while the increased blood flow to the brain that occurs during REM sleep may be necessary for mental health. At different times in our life we seem to need more or less of each type of sleep, but because we have no control over the type of sleep we get, we can only try to ensure that we get enough total sleep to meet our needs.

Natural rhythms and health

The combined action of natural rhythms and external time-givers help us to live in harmony with our environment. When we go to bed at a regular time at night and get up at a regular time in the morning, we are acting in harmony with nature, and generally sleep better as a result. The pre-programming of body rhythms and associated physiological processes to external signals also allows us to prepare for sleep at night, a natural process that enables us to relax and become more inclined to snuggle up in the warmth as darkness approaches. Likewise, the demands of morning are met by increases in body temperature and hormonal activity giving us a warm up and wake-up call, all of which is helped along by stimulating daylight. In short, our body rhythms do not react to our environment, but act in accordance with it, anticipating change and enabling us to meet its demands.

Sleep changes and illness
One British survey of 9,000 people showed a direct relationship between days taken off work due to illness and changes in sleep habits.

Chapter Three

Duration and pattern of sleep

Shakespeare called sleep "the chief nourisher of life's feast". The metaphor works well, because sleep, like food, is an essential, but easily abused ingredient in life. In the quest for healing sleep it is tempting to think that the longer you sleep the better for your health. The belief that good sleep consists of an uninterrupted eight hours of slumber is one that is firmly entrenched in our culture. Those who manage only five hours a night, or find it difficult to get by on less than ten, often feel abnormal. Sleep needs, like appetite and taste, are a very individual matter.

How much sleep do we need?

It is accepted that two thirds of the adult population sleep for an average seven and a half hours a night. About 16 per cent sleep more than eight and a half hours and 16 per cent sleep less than six and a half hours. When you consider that a survey taken in 1910 showed that healthy young adults slept for an average of nine hours a night, it may seem that our need for sleep is in decline. However, some experts suggest that for many people the average is not enough. Researchers at the North Valley Sleep Disorder Center in California claim about half of us are not getting enough sleep. British sleep specialist Dr Jim Horne believes in quality over quantity. He maintains that six hours is more than enough for good health and anything more than that is optional. Dr Horne suggests that what we need is what he calls "core sleep" – a combination of deep, slow-wave sleep and REM sleep, which are the restful and restoring stages of sleep. Research has

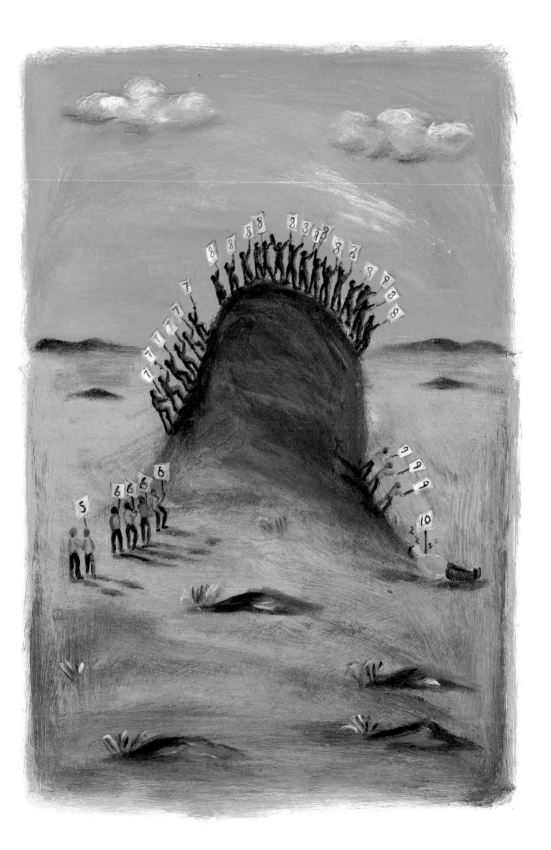

shown that short sleepers can get as much core sleep as those who sleep longer, because they dispense with much of the "optional", light sleep and fill the time with the more important types of sleep.

Evolution seems to have had an influence on how much optional sleep we take. Our relatively safe existence means we can sleep for much longer, free from the threat of dangerous predators. This is a pattern that is repeated in the animal kingdom. Animals that are seldom attacked sleep for much longer and more deeply than those whose popularity with meat-eaters requires them to be continuously vigilant against attack.

The consequences of lack of sleep

An obsession with clocking up hours of sleep is likely to be more damaging than missing an hour of slumber. Losing a few hours sleep occasionally is not believed to be damaging to health, it simply makes you feel tired and slightly irritable. Whatever sleep you lose one day, will be compensated for the following day. This ability of the human body to be self-regulating means that in an ideal world, we should all get enough sleep. However, our world is far from ideal and aggravating factors such as stress, irregular hours, illness, and excessive noise means that some people regularly go without the amount of sleep they need.

One of the immediate consequences of sleep deprivation is poor concentration and lack of judgement. So people who sleep badly run a greater risk of accidental injury when driving or operating dangerous machinery. They also make poor decisions and frequent mistakes. Constant tiredness can also lead to irritability, memory loss, depression, and stress. Feeling stressed and anxious about not sleeping means you sleep even less, so you may get in a cycle of fatigue and sleeplessness that is hard to break. The familiar visible effects of insufficient sleep include dark circles under the eyes and unhealthy skin.

In the long term, the body's defence systems may be

Sleep and personality
Personality is believed to play a part in determining sleep needs. Short sleepers are characterized as hard-working extroverts, who are energetic, ambitious, and confident. Long sleepers are supposed to be worriers, who are less self-assured, non-conformist, mildly neurotic, but also more creative and artistic. The French poet Voltaire is believed to have needed only three hours sleep a night and Britain's ex-prime minister Margaret Thatcher boasted of similar needs. But the scientific genius, Albert Einstein, is reputed to have slept for 12 hours at a stretch.

affected. Studies have shown that when healthy young adults are deprived of sleep for even one or two days they produce fewer natural killer cells (the white blood cells that fight infection) and so have a lowered resistance to infections such as colds and flu.

Research has also shown that people naturally enjoy more deep, slow-wave sleep when recovering from illness or an operation and this speeds up the healing process. People recovering from serious conditions in intensive care units demonstrate how sleep deprivation may inhibit healing. In intensive care units lights are on day and night, noise and activity continue throughout the night, and the need for frequent medical intervention make undisturbed sleep an impossibility. All of this contributes to a condition known as "intensive care unit syndrome", in which recovery is slowed, and the patient experiences mental stress, often becoming deluded and paranoid. When normal sleep patterns are resumed these symptoms are resolved.

Too much sleep

Sleep deprivation studies suggest we need at least two hours' sleep a day, but no more than 15. We appear to have an inbuilt alarm clock that stops us from sleeping too long. When sleep-deprived volunteers and sponsored "wakathon" participants were allowed to sleep indefinitely, none of them slept continuously for longer than 15 hours. These people had stayed awake for days on end yet they paid off their "sleep debt" in one long night. If you miss a night's sleep you do not need two nights of long sleep to make up for it. It usually takes only an extra hour or two to make up the deficit. In fact, several years ago researchers in California showed that having a long lie in or sleeping at irregular times could cause the same feelings of irritability and lead to the same sort of incompetence as lack of sleep. This confirms the view expressed in traditional Chinese medicine that too much sleep is as unhealthy as too little, and that both problems are a sign of imbalance.

Sleep needs through life

Our sleep needs change throughout life – both in terms of the total amount of sleep needed and the times at which it is taken. Children have different needs from adults and adults of differing ages or stages of life also have individual needs. The length and quality of sleep is also influenced by factors other than age – for example, women's sleep is affected by hormonal changes. What many people see as a sleep problem may simply be a normal response to natural changes in life.

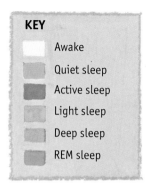

KEY

Awake

Quiet sleep

Active sleep

Light sleep

Deep sleep

REM sleep

Childhood sleep patterns

Newborn babies can sleep for a total of 16 to 18 hours a day. Young babies often go straight from wakefulness to REM sleep (termed active sleep in this age group), cutting out stages one to four (termed quiet sleep in this age group). As they get older babies sleep less, but for much longer periods at a time. By the age of three or four a child spends about three hours a night in deep sleep, three to four hours in REM sleep, and just under five hours in light sleep. The amount of REM sleep decreases to the normal adult quota of about two hours a night by the age of ten.

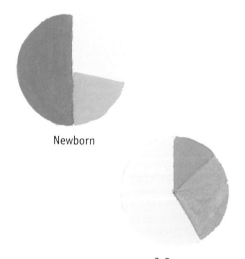

Newborn

3-5 years

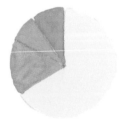

13-15 years

The teenage years

During adolescence the need for sleep temporarily increases The amount of deep sleep decreases between the ages of 11 and 17 but the overall need for sleep increases. Given the opportunity, an adolescent can easily clock up ten hours of sleep a night. The fact that those in their mid to late teens can get a full night's sleep and still become sleepy during the daytime adds to evidence that this is a time when more sleep is essential.

From adulthood to middle age

Adults between the ages of 20 and 30 have relatively stable sleep patterns. Twenty-year-olds have an average of seven and a half hours' sleep a night, consisting of just under an hour and a half of deep sleep, nearly four hours of light sleep, and about two hours of REM sleep. Sleep patterns begin to change around 40 to 45 years of age in men and 50 to 55 in women.

20-29 years

70-79 years

Later years

After middle age the amount of deep sleep gradually reduces. Most people over the age of 70 sleep for less than seven hours a night. In this age group only 23 minutes is spent in deep sleep. The vast majority of sleep is light and frequently disrupted.

Individual requirements

In otherwise healthy people sleep can be affected by the following:

♦ *Inborn traits.* Some babies and children naturally do not need much sleep, and tend to grow into adults who need little sleep.

♦ *Exercise and metabolism.* People who get more exercise during the day enjoy sound sleep at night. This isprobably linked to the rise in body temperature produced by exercise, which seems to promote deep sleep. This may also explain why people with a high metabolic rate seem to get more deep sleep than other body types.

♦ *Serious long term weight loss.* This lowers body temperature and has a damaging effect on sleep.

Women's special needs

Hormonal changes can affect the quantity and quality of women's sleep. Women who suffer with pre-menstrual syndrome tend to get less REM sleep and deep sleep in the pre-menstrual period than those who do not. As a result they do not get the quality of sleep they need and may feel extra tired and irritable at that time.

During the first three months of pregnancy women are frequently tired and desperate for naps during the day. Researchers at the University of California have found that this could possibly be explained by the fact that pregnant women tend to get less deep sleep and have more sleep disruptions. This may be due to increased levels of the hormone progesterone.

The menopause can also be a time of sleep disruption as a result of hot flushes and night sweats. However, the menopause has some positive effects. Research suggests that menopausal changes may help to ensure that women get sufficient amounts of deep sleep. Women get their full quota of deep sleep for ten years longer than men. The fact that women tend to live longer than men has been attributed in part to this extra helping of deep sleep.

Sleep patterns: nature or nurture?

Sleep may be a natural state, but when we sleep is a matter of convention. This is not as contradictory as it seems. After all many of our natural functions are controlled by convention: eating is natural, yet we train ourselves to eat at particular times; urinating is natural, yet as children we all have to be toilet-trained. Sleeping is what is known as a modified innate activity, meaning we do it instinctively, but we need to learn when to do it acceptably.

Babies sleep whenever they want because nobody makes any demands on their time. Parents teach their children to go to sleep when they are put to bed and they gradually develop a pattern of sleeping that is socially acceptable. Bad sleep habits developed in childhood are very hard to break. Childhood sleep problems are discussed in more detail in Chapter Seven.

Siestas, naps, and microsleeps

In some cultures, particularly in the Mediterranean, an afternoon siesta is the norm. There is evidence to suggest that an afternoon nap that does not interfere with night sleep can improve mood, concentration, and productivity. Our body rhythms indicate a natural inclination to sleep during the mid afternoon, and some sleep experts believe a short afternoon nap could be all it takes to restore flagging energy levels, sharpen mental performance, and eliminate many of the problems associated with midday fatigue. Unfortunately, most people's lifestyles do not allow for an afternoon siesta. Those who can manage it tend to be people working from home or older people who have retired.

Shiftworkers and people who sleep badly at night may feel tempted to nap whenever they get the chance. Napping allows you to catch up on your sleep but it does not provide a long-term solution to a sleeping problem. It may simply perpetuate the cycle of staying awake at night.

Ayurvedic practitioners believe that naps can be beneficial, but only if you decide to take a nap and not if you are
suddenly overwhelmed by sleep. Deepak Chopra claims
"the notion of intention is a fundamental part of the
action. If intention is not present the benefits of napping
are nullified." Naps are intended as light refreshment, not
a substitute for sleep. They should not last longer than
30 minutes, otherwise you go into deep sleep, from which
it may be hard to wake up and you are likely to feel worse
than when you went to sleep.

Older people, who sleep less during the night, often
experience brief periods of sleep in the day lasting for
a matter of seconds, known as microsleeps. These have the
same refreshing effect as brief periods of normal sleep, but
may reduce the amount of sleep needed at night. Studies
in sleep laboratories show that 25 per cent of 70-year-olds
and 45 per cent of 80-year-olds nap during the day.

> **A normal night's sleep?**
> Dr Chris Idzikowski, Chair
> of the British Sleep Society,
> claims that asking how much
> sleep we need is like asking
> how fast we should breathe.
> It depends on what we have
> been doing while awake and
> is mostly beyond our control.

Accepting your own sleep needs

Many people who think they have insomnia are unaware
that they simply need less sleep. We are all individuals
with individual needs and while some of us need nine
hours of undisturbed slumber, others can spring out of
bed after five. However, what we do need to do is recognize
our sleep needs. If you are naturally a short sleeper and
feel well during the day in spite of little sleep, relax and
enjoy the fact that you have more time to enjoy yourself.
It is healthier to live according to your natural sleep patterns than to feel stressed about not sleeping "normally".
If you go to bed and habitually lie awake for an hour
every night wondering why you can't get to sleep, try
going to bed an hour later or getting up an hour earlier
and see what happens. You may find you sleep better
and generally become less anxious. However, if you are
constantly tired and feel that you really need more sleep,
but for some reason are not getting it, then you would
be well-advised to take a closer look at your daily routine
and all aspects of your lifestyle.

Chapter Four

The role of dreams

It's impossible to know if our prehistoric ancestors woke from nightmarish confrontations with ravening beasts or dreams of victory over club-wielding neighbours, but the chances are they did. For as long as humans have been documenting history, we have been documenting dreams and attempting to fathom their significance. Yet we still know relatively little about dreams and their significance in our lives.

We spend about a quarter of each night in a dream world, which means that in an average lifetime we spend about six years dreaming. Yet, in many ways the whole area of dreaming remains as much a mystery today as it was in ancient times. What is clear from laboratory research is that everybody dreams. Some people claim they never dream, but scientists have shown that these "non-dreamers" simply forget their dreams very quickly or believe that they were only thinking in their sleep.

Traditional and modern views

Throughout history different cultures have produced their own explanations for the phenomenon of dreaming. Many traditional societies past and present have believed that dreams could be used to predict the future, to sort out psychological problems and, most importantly, to contact supernatural figures and learn or receive special powers from them. Some cultures, such as those of the native Americans, have valued dream experiences to the extent that they tried to encourage the right dreams by fasting, meditating, and choosing special places in which

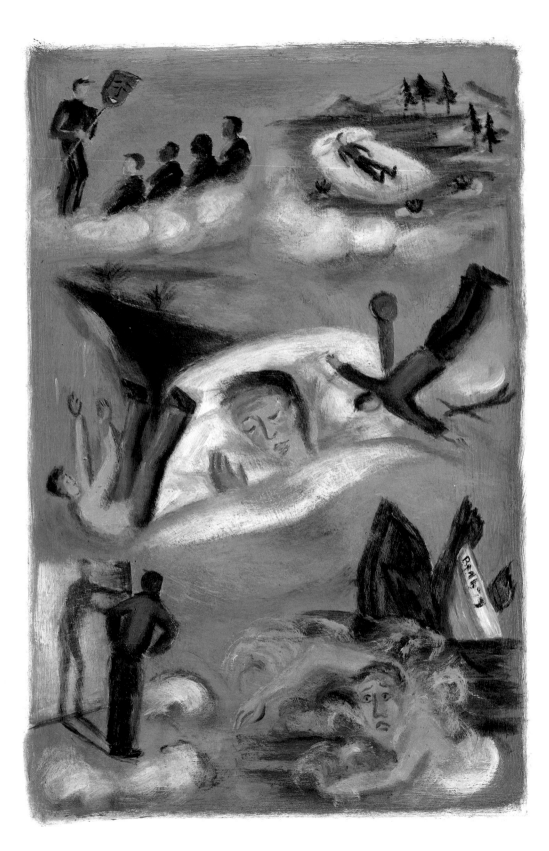

to sleep. In these societies there was a clear assumption that dreams could have an influence on waking life. By confronting danger they became braver, by listening to the spirits they became wiser, and by sleeping on a problem they could find an answer.

Central to native American dream theory was the concept of a guide, an entity who would guide the dreamer safely through the world of sleep and help the dreamer to bring back wisdom. Shamans (medicine men and women or witchdoctors) used dreams to wander in the spirit world and learn the secrets of the dead. Dreams were also used to facilitate personal transformation. A person who fought and died in a dream, could be spiritually reborn as a better, stronger, wiser person.

In most eastern philosophical and medical traditions people are not viewed simply as a body controlled by a mind, but as a complex integration of mind, body, and spirit. The spiritual dimension is the aspect of dreaming on which most eastern traditions focus. For example, Tibetan Buddhists use dreams as a way of communing with the soul. To die while dreaming means the dream will continue.

Modern psychologists are divided in their opinions about our need to dream. Many believe that dreaming is essential for a healthy, well-developed, and efficient brain in the same way that deep sleep is necessary for physical health, growth, and restoration. This seems a plausible explanation. Most dreaming occurs during REM sleep and people denied REM sleep become irritable, moody, and tired, and frequently suffer from impaired memory and concentration.

At a purely functional level dreams appear to perform the task of clearing out and organizing the mental clutter that accumulates during the day. This appears to keep us mentally alert and balanced, and capable of concentrating and learning during the day. A mental spring clean may also clear the mind of distractions and thereby allow it to explore the subconscious.

> "Nature doesn't do anything for nothing. If the purpose of sleep is indeed to restore the body, we must account for the fact that during a significant portion of our sleep time this restoration isn't accomplished simply through passive rest. Instead, a positive, creative process is taking place that requires significant energy."
>
> **Deepak Chopra**
> *Restful Sleep*

The interpretation of dreams

Dreams are thoughts and images that occur during sleep, forming a complex internal response to external events. They spring from our subconscious, where there are no boundaries between past, future, and present and where logic loses its grip.

Mythology, cultural, and individual beliefs have as much to offer on dream interpretation as psychology. Most cultures in the world also have a history of belief in the spiritual significance of dreams. Good dreams were commonly believed to carry messages from the gods or God and bad dreams were sent by evil spirits. Many societies developed their own systems of dream interpretation. In contrast, western scientists and psychologists tend to disregard the spiritual aspects of dreams as myth. Before the development of psychoanalysis, most scientists and doctors considered dreams to be little more than mental garbage. Some people still subscribe to this theory, but others believe that dreams serve a more purposeful role in maintaining mental and spiritual health.

All systems of dream interpretation rely heavily on symbolism. In dreams, not everything is as it seems. Dictionaries of dream symbolism frequently offer "definitions" of symbols. But when you flick through three or four of these volumes, it soon becomes obvious that there is no definitive guide to dream interpretation. There are certain classic symbols such as houses, people, flying, and appearing naked, on which there is general agreement. But ultimately dreams are a personal journey and their content is best interpreted by the dreamer.

> "dream research is one of the few remaining areas where the layperson is as competent as the professional."
>
> **Dr David Fontana**
> *The Secret Language of Dreams*

The Freudian view

The undisputed father of modern western dream analysis was the Czechoslovakian-born psychologist Sigmund Freud (1856-1939). Freud claimed that "the interpretation of dreams is the royal road to a knowledge of the unconscious activities of the mind".

Freud saw the mind as being divided into the subconscious, which he called the "id" – a place of chaos, base urges, and amorality – and the conscious mind, called the "ego", which imposes order and reason on our thoughts. Our conscience, the judge of good and evil, he called the "super ego". He suggested that during our waking life the ego maintains order and morality in our minds and suppresses the desires of the id. During sleep, however, the ego relaxes its control and the id makes its desires known through dreams. He believed these desires could be so disturbing and potentially damaging that the ego censored the more disruptive elements and presented them to the dreamer in the form of symbols. The symbolism of dreams held the key to unlocking the secrets of the subconscious. In recent years Freud has fallen out of favour, but his work remains of monumental significance in the world of dream analysis.

The Jungian view

The Swiss psychologist Carl Jung (1875-1961) initially worked closely with Freud before they parted company in 1913. Jung developed his own branch of psychology called analytical psychology, which was heavily influenced by myth, mysticism, religion, metaphysics, and symbol. He concluded that common psychological themes spanned the ages and the cultures of the world, and that we all possess both consciousness and personal unconscious, which roughly related to Freud's ego and id. Instead of the censorious super ego, he believed in the existence of a collective unconscious.

For Jung the collective unconscious was the deepest area of the mind, a sort of common psychological pool that was dipped into by everyone in the world. He termed dreams that stemmed from this collective unconscious "grand dreams", which he saw as giving us access to "the vast historical storehouse of the human race". Jung believed dreams were the key to discovering and exploring the higher levels of consciousness, spirituality,

Major Jungian archetypes

Jung belived that certain "primordial images" hold symbolic meaning for us all and can be used to interpret dreams. The appearance of one or more of these archetypal images in a dream, according to Jungian thought, holds a universal significance.

The persona

The image we present to the world, not our "real self". It appears in dreams as a figure. If we confuse persona and real self, it can appear as an undesirable figure. Being naked in a dream can symbolize loss of persona.

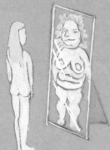

The shadow

The instinctive, or weaker side of our nature. It provokes negative reactions such as fear and anger. Its appearance in dreams can suggest we need to exercise more control over our weaknesses.

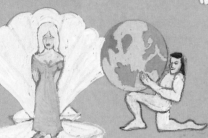

The anima and animus

The feminine and masculine aspects of everyone's personality. The anima is the feminine qualities in men, often represented by a beautiful or goddess-like figure. The animus is the masculine qualities in women, represented by a god-like, heroic, or powerful man.

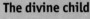

The divine child

The child within, a symbol of the true self. The appearance of a baby or child in a dream suggests vulnerability, but also freshness, spontaneity, and potential. Making contact with the child can put us in touch with our true self.

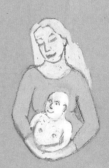

The wise old man

A father, priest, teacher, or other figure of authority. In a man's dream the wise old man can represent the self. But he is also seen as a "mana" personality, a powerful figure who could guide us towards the higher self, but also has the ability to lead us away from it.

The great mother

A symbol of growth, nurturing and fertility, but also of seduction, possession, and dominance. The great mother appears in many forms: as a mother, priestess, or princess or as a witch, seductress or terrible mother.

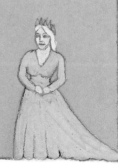

and love. Jung claimed that the collective unconscious was made up of "primordial images, innate in the human mind" which he called archetypes. Understanding the archetypes would enable us to understand the language of our dreams and to distinguish personal dreams from those of universal significance. Some of the archetypes are described on p.47.

Recent developments in dream interpretation

Much of modern dream interpretation is still based on the pioneering work of Freud and Jung, but it is also influenced by the work of American psychiatrist Fritz Perls (1893-1970) the father of Gestalt therapy. Perls thought that the symbols were a product of our own experience. He also thought that every character in our dreams represented aspects of our self that we may not acknowledge when awake. He considered dreams to be representative of emotional unfinished business, with which we had to deal. Our dream symbolism was the personal vocabulary of each dreamer's mind and not of universal significance.

The Swiss psychiatrist Medard Boss (b.1903), suggested that dreams could usually be interpreted on a literal, rather than a symbolic level. For Boss there is no universal morality on which we can draw, a dream simply reveals the dreamer's beliefs, behaviour, and relationships.

Some psychologists less enamoured of the idea of dream interpretation favour the idea that during sleep the brain produces bursts of random sensory information that the brain tries to process by weaving into some sort of story. The brain uses the hopes and fears of the dreamer to help compile the dream story. A similar theory suggests that during sleep the brain creates a story that accommodates all the events, thoughts, and activities of the previous day and processes them in such a way that enables us to store them in the memory. In other words, a dream is a memory aid. Another theory compares the brain to a computer in which dreams are a means of filing away largely unnecessary information to make space for the information we need on a day-to-day basis.

The Ayurvedic view

Ayurvedic texts associate dream themes with the three *doshas*. A sudden change in the type of dream you have been having can indicate a doshic imbalance. For example, if your dreams suddenly take on *pitta* qualities, they can indicate an increase in *pitta* energies. According to Ayurveda, dreams are believed to be both a reaction to the events of the day and an expression of unfulfilled desires, and dream symbolism can be either personal or universal – a concept on which both Freud and Jung agreed.

The traditional Chinese approach

In Chinese philosophy dream analysis is an integral part of medical diagnosis. Dreams that do not frighten you, disturb your sleep, or leave you feeling mentally unsettled the next morning are considered normal. But nightmares or dreams which leave you feeling tired are believed to be "excessive" and the product of a pathological condition.

Traditional Chinese medicine sees the person as a combination of different types of energy. Energy is distributed throughout the body by a system of meridians, a network of invisible channels. The type of dream that an individual experiences is governed by the balance of energy in organs and meridians. For example, a dream of building a house is a sign of spleen deficiency, which can manifest as weight problems and fatigue.

According to the Chinese tradition, each hour of the day and night relates to a different organ and emotion. The time that your dream takes place is an important guide to its significance. For example, the hours of 3 to 5am – the start of the spiritual day – relate to the lungs and sadness or grief. Dreams that occur during this time may cause breathing difficulties or deal with feelings of loss, and may be of a spiritual nature.

Ayurvedic dream themes

Vata types are believed to have imaginative, active dreams, and when this *dosha* is imbalanced it can cause dreams of anxiety. In *vata* types anxiety tends to be expressed in dreams of movement such as falling, being chased, or trying to run away.

Pitta types tend to have dreams of action and adventure. When *pitta* is out of balance, these can turn to dreams of anger and conflict.

Kaphas are believed to have very tranquil dreams that they rarely remember. It is typically *kapha* to dream of lakes or oceans, for example.

What your dreams reveal

The content of our dreams may provide insights into how we subconsciously handle life experiences. Interpretation is largely subjective. When you start to investigate your dreams, you may find recurrent themes or images that relate to events in your life or state of mind. These themes may be significant only for you, but they can also have a more universal relevance. Some of the emotions or situations that can provoke vivid dreams are described on the following pages along with classic examples of the dream imagery that psychologists have identified as subconscious expressions of those emotions.

Anxiety

Anxiety is commonly expressed by dreams of falling, drowning, or being chased or trying to run away while feeling rooted to the spot. Sometimes the dreams reveal the nature of the anxiety. For example, a dream of trying to finish a never-ending job may suggest a problem of overwork. Some people find that a particular dream recurs at times of stress. Those who have long since finished taking exams may still dream of sitting an exam for which they have not revised.

Change and identity

Major life changes such as moving house or marriage may have an impact on the unconscious mind. Well-recognized symbols of change include crossing bridges or doorsteps. Dreams of altering your appearance or that of your home may indicate life changes and their effect on your identity. Being lost in an unfamiliar landscape is often a sign of anxiety about a move. However, being lost in a fog, a maze, or a web of confusing streets may also signify a loss of direction in life. Feelings of sadness about changes in dreams may indicate unreadiness for a real-life change. Whereas feeling happy can suggest the reverse.

Repressed feelings

Dreams of violence towards those close to you can indicate repressed feelings of anger. Some psychologists would interpret the violence as a desire to attack the source of your distressing feelings rather than kill or harm that person.

Happiness

Happy dreams may focus on pleasurable experiences or well-recognized symbols of good luck, but they can also be filled with more abstract symbolism such as bright light, vibrant colours, or a sensation of wonder. Traditionally light relates to spiritual enlightenment. Dreaming of a rainbow, a Judeo-Christian symbol of hope, is widely believed to signify good luck. Among Australian aboriginal peoples the rainbow is a sign of spiritual transformation.

Success and failure

Examples of dreams related to success include winning a race, scaling a wall, or winning a fight or prize. Actually overcoming an obstacle in a dream may show that you have the confidence to overcome whatever stands between you and success. Dreaming of talking to people who cannot hear you suggests feelings of inadequacy and fear of failure. Other similar dreams include knocking on a door that nobody answers and being invisible. Although dreams of success and failure may relate to actual events, more often they are indicative of the dreamer's state of mind.

Death and grief

In dream symbolism death can be interpreted as the end of a phase and is therefore a positive sign of rebirth. Grief not expressed in waking life can find an outlet in dreams. It is not uncommon to dream of a dead friend or relative. Such dreams can leave you comforted or distraught depending on the atmosphere and events of the dream. They may be pleasantly nostalgic, which can be healing. Dreams in which the deceased is not really dead but trapped or buried alive, or is angry with you, or trying to get back home, can be distressing, but releasing those thoughts through dreams can play a part in the healthy expression of grief.

Sex

Dreams about sex are common, especially during adolescence. Frequent sexual dreams may indicate a high sex drive, or simply be a sign of sexual frustration. Sex, of course, occupies a great part of our waking thoughts, and our conscious thoughts naturally filter into our dreams in either explicit or muted forms. Freudian psychologists tend to see sex in any rhythmic activity such as riding a horse or rowing a boat. Certain symbols are also given sexual significance: a knife is believed to represent the penis, while a purse can represent the female reproductive organs. Carl Jung believed that even explicit sexual dreams could be interpreted on a higher creative level.

Spirituality

Flying unaided can be seen as symbolic of soaring above reality or of reaching the higher self. In many cultures there is a belief in astral travel (an out-of-body dream experience). African and aboriginal shamans claim to receive their calling in dreams where they fly through the air or meet with spirits. The experience of astral travel is believed to be similar to when the soul leaves the body at death, except that during dreams we are tied to the physical body by means of a silver cord, which is severed at death. Climbing of any kind is also seen as spiritual progress.

Dreams and waking life

Dreams may not only be a product of the emotional content of our waking lives, but the emotional experiences of our dreams may in fact influence our conscious existence. For example, the Senoi people of Malaysia encourage healthy emotional development in their children by teaching them to become actively involved in their dreams. They learn to become courageous by confronting danger in their dreams and they become wise by listening to dream advisers.

Dream emotions produce real physiological changes. Vivid dreams can cause heart rate and breathing to become irregular and increase the production of gastric acid, producing similar physical effects to conscious anxiety, fear, anger, and excitement. Learning to conquer fear or experience bliss in dreams can enable us to do likewise in real life, encouraging healthy emotional responses.

A third level of consciousness

The fact that REM sleep is notably different from either NREM sleep or wakefulness also suggests that what occurs during REM sleep has a special function. In fact some American sleep researchers claim that REM sleep is neither sleep nor wakefulness, but a third distinct form of human existence. Research appears to have led them to a conclusion similar to one Ayurvedic seers arrived at thousands of years ago. They claimed that human consciousness consists of several layers, including waking, dreamless sleep, dreaming, and the joy that comes with enlightenment. This idea that dreaming is actually a third level of consciousness may help to explain the concept of using dreams to explore mental and physical health and as a key to the spiritual world. It is possible that all dreams contain something of value, if only we could remember and understand them. We may have lost the ability to use

Sleep learning

In the 1960s many people believed sleep to be a waste of valuable learning time, so they used the time to learn from instruction tapes, while still asleep. Results were disappointing as any information learnt faded as quickly as a dream. Sleep learning was also found to prevent spontaneous dreaming and interfere with concentration levels during the day.

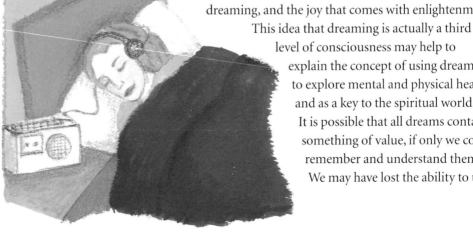

dreams, but this is a skill that can be re-learned. Many people have turned to the wisdom of ancient traditions, such as Buddhism and the native American tradition, in order to learn how to work with dreams. Increasingly people in the West are beginning to trust in the power of the subconscious and use it to improve mental and physical health, and to gain control over their lives. Hypnosis, which taps the power of the subconscious and uses it to shut out pain, fight disease, and even stimulate cell renewal, is one way in which many people have learnt to use this vast untapped resource.

Inventive dreams

Elias Howe the man who invented the sewing machine is reputed to have been baffled as to where to put the hole for the thread. One night he dreamt of Africans throwing spears. In the tip of each spear was an eye-shaped hole. When he woke up Elias knew exactly where to put the hole in his needle.

Dreams and illness

The ancient Greek belief that dreams could reveal important information about the state of our health is not only echoed in traditional eastern beliefs, it has also found favour with modern dream researchers. The fact that REM sleep is a time of changes in breathing, heart rate, and other physiological consequences of stress has lead some researchers to conclude that there could be a link between dreaming and stress-related illness. Studies have suggested that dreams can in some cases alert the dreamer to the presence of organic disease, trigger disease, or indicate the development of psychosomatic illness.

Night-time attacks of migraine and asthma have been linked with REM sleep. Respiratory and heart problems have been shown to occur after dreams, particularly dreams of an emotional nature. People with duodenal ulcers have been found to secrete more gastric acid during sleep than those who do not have an ulcer.

Research has also shown that certain dream themes indicate the presence of different illnesses. Dreams of death and dying in men and dreams of separation (such as divorce or being separated from her child) in women indicate the presence of organic disease, especially heart disease. Dreams of terror relate to migraine, and dreams of lost resources have been shown to indicate dementia. One study showed that people who claimed they never dreamed had the highest mortality rate of all. These studies have led some researchers to conclude that dreams may come to warn us of physical or mental illness, but they disappear when illness becomes critical.

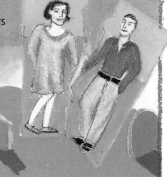

Using your dreams

Tibetan Buddhists believe that by developing our spirituality we can exert control over our dreams and learn from them. Some Buddhist teachers and students are reputed to be so enlightened that they can appear to each other in dreams to discuss issues of importance. The next morning both people know what was discussed in the dream. Among the native American peoples the determination of the dreamer was considered vital to successful dream experiences. If you wanted a particular type of information or guidance you had to will that you would get it. Concentration was enhanced by fasting, meditation, prayer, and isolation. Modern sleep research confirms that these elements may well enhance our dreaming abilities. A day filled with quietness and contemplation, can double our normal quantity of REM sleep and possibly produce richer dreams.

Problem solving

The traditional belief that sleeping on a problem can help to resolve it suggests that we can use dreams at both a literal and symbolic level, to sort out issues that defy conscious efforts. If you have been wrestling with an issue that makes you anxious and disturbs your sleep, then it needs to be resolved and your dreams may be the place to do it. Psychologists who believe that the subconscious mind carries on working on a problem when you have consciously forgotten about it, call this process "incubation". Many people who work with dreams believe that we can learn to use these incubated ideas to our advantage.

One famous example of successful dream problem solving is that of the German scientist Friedrich Kekulé who discovered the "benzene ring" in a dream. Kekulé, who had been trying desperately to understand the molecular structure of benzene, fell asleep and dreamt of molecules dancing before his eyes. The molecules kept forming into different patterns and finally joined up to form a ring – the solution to his problem!

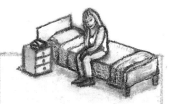

How to encourage problem-solving dreams

♦ Study the problem during the day and tell yourself that you will find a solution.

♦ If the problem keeps cropping up during the day, tell yourself not to worry because you will find an answer in your dreams.

♦ Go to bed with a clear image of the problem and tell your mind that you want an answer.

♦ When you wake up record your dream immediately.

♦ The dream message may not always be clear, but record all the images. By following clues and associations you may be able to arrive at a solution.

Lucid dreams

Lucid dreaming is a state in which you are aware that you are dreaming and use that awareness to control your dream. It has been claimed that spiritually advanced people can retain conscious control of their dreams in this way and that doing so can be enormously valuable in terms of learning and spiritual growth. Lucid dreams tend to seem more real than other types of dreaming and our senses of smell, taste, sound, and sight are more keen. Some masters of the technique are believed to be able to visit other people in their dreams to advise or comfort them. Dream therapists claim that with patience and practice we can all learn to retain some conscious control over our dream events. The key is to develop a better knowledge of your own mind by learning to distinguish between conscious and unconscious thought. Research has shown that lucid dreamers seem to be less neurotic and depressive than non lucid dreamers.

How to encourage lucid dreaming

♦ Meditation improves concentration and will help you to recognize when you are in a dream. Becoming more aware of what is real will also help you recognize a dream world.

♦ Throughout the day test yourself on how you know you are not dreaming now, for example, by noting that people do not fly or change into monsters or that if you want to run you will not feel glued to the spot.

♦ As you drift off to sleep tell yourself repeatedly, "I know when I am dreaming" and picture yourself as an observer of your own dream.

♦ Record your dreams. When you begin to recognize when you are dreaming you can begin to use your dreams to your own advantage.

Prophetic dreams

Dreams that predict the future may fall into the category of "big" dreams, meaning they are dreams that can have significance for an entire community, or they may be "little" dreams, having significance only for the dreamer. According to dream researchers, it is quite common to dream of events waiting to happen and the subconscious mind can access these events in the same way as it can glean information from the past. Occasionally we hear of people who have dreamt of a disaster about to happen or the location of a missing person. Many of these people say they "see" the event as if it were already front page news. Researchers at the Maimonides Dream Laboratory in New York found astonishingly positive results when they tested the accuracy of precognitive dreams.

Dreams of past lives

A belief in reincarnation is common in cultures where dreams are valued. Dream workers who believe in reincarnation claim that the soul can access the skills and knowledge of past lives through the subconscious. Past-life therapy is used by some to treat physical and psychological ailments which they believe were caused in a previous life. However, dreams of past lives are not necessarily evidence of the dreamer having lived before, they may simply be information that the dreamer has gleaned from dipping into the collective unconscious. Whatever your personal beliefs, the dreams can be beneficial. People who claim to have had past-life dreams say that these dreams can offer explicit and dramatic explanations for the dreamer's recurrent aches, pains, illnesses, or fears.

Nightmares

Everyone knows what it is like to have a bad dream. Traditionally thought of as visitations from evil spirits, nightmares are now more commonly thought of as expressions of anxiety or repressed feelings of fear, guilt, or grief. Many people have nightmares after a particularly traumatic event in their lives. Drugs and alcohol can also trigger nightmares. In children common causes are anxieties about school or family life. Television programmes, frightening stories, and more serious issues such as separation, neglect, and abuse, can also be to blame.

Nightmares often force us to confront issues with which we have refused to deal and they contain a message that demands to be heard. If the subconscious is trying so desperately to attract our attention to a particular issue, it may be more healthy to deal with it rather than shy away from it. Psychologist David Fontana says that we can use nightmares to our advantage when we recognize that the fear they cause lies in our reaction to them rather than anything intrinsically evil in the dream. People who have recurrent nightmares may find that working with the nightmares can help to bring them to an end.

Dealing with nightmares

♦ By interpreting symbols, try to find out how the content of your dream relates to your own fears or emotions.

♦ If you experience a series of nightmares look for a link and try to decipher the subconscious message.

♦ Strip the nightmare of its fear by learning to confront danger in your dreams. Tell your mind before you go to sleep that dream characters cannot harm you and that you will stand up to anything that chases or attacks you.

♦ A child who dreams of a monster can learn to handle the fear by drawing the monster in a cage.

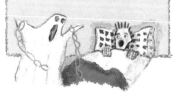

Recording your dreams

If you want to use your dreams, you need to record them. Some people never remember their dreams and many more of us forget them soon after we wake up. Even dreams that are vivid on waking fade throughout the day. This may be because certain dreams are just too distressing to remember. Another theory is that the sleeping state prevents us from remembering in the normal way. Devotees of dream interpretation, however, claim that it is possible to remember as many as five dreams a night.

Keeping a dream diary

People even briefly distracted first thing in the morning quickly forget their dreams. Set your alarm and make your diary your first priority. Date each dream and note your feelings as well as the dream details. Drawing is a more spontaneous exercise than marshalling your thoughts into prose. Sketching the dream images may therefore be the best way to capture the essence of the dream. You will probably need to record numerous dreams before you can begin to find common themes.

Dream diary checklist

Record all the events of your dream in the order in which they appeared.

♦ Detail all the characters (including animals) in your dream. Who were they? What did they do or say? What did they look like? Were they fantasy characters?

♦ Write down the precise content of any dream conversations.

♦ Make a note of the dream setting. Did the scenery seem real or fantastical? If it was a familiar place such as your kitchen, was it an exact reproduction of your kitchen?

♦ List all objects, signs, and symbols, real and imaginary, and note the colours in your dreams.

♦ Describe the atmosphere of the dream and how it affected you. Note any changes of mood and how you felt when you woke up.

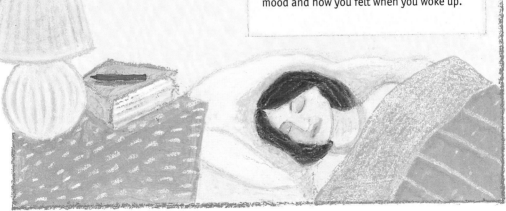

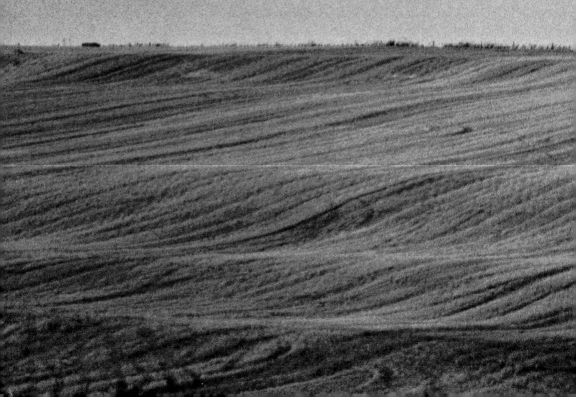

PART TWO

The world of sleeplessness

O sleep! O gentle sleep!
Nature's soft nurse, how have I frighted thee,
That thou no more wilt weigh
mine eyelids down…

William Shakespeare
1564-1616

Chapter Five

The enemies of sleep

The human body is designed to sleep through the night, so that we can be creative and productive during the day, but in the "developed" societies of the late 20th century instead of experiencing regularly alternating periods of energy-giving sunlight and restful darkness, we are exposed to the unremitting glare of artificial light throughout the day and night. We work long, and often irregular hours, and stress keeps our bodies in a perpetual state of alertness, often unrelieved by the release of physical exertion. Add to all of this, noise pollution, bad diet, smoking, over-consumption of alcohol, lack of exercise, and it becomes surprising that we sleep at all.

Understanding the causes of sleeplessness

There is no doubt that how we live affects how well we sleep. The factors in a daily routine that contribute to sleep are known collectively as "sleep hygiene". Improvements in sleep hygiene can make a remarkable difference to the quality of sleep, but will not necessary solve a chronic problem. Sleep disorders are only rarely caused by external factors alone. For example, noise may be the immediate cause of your waking at night, but worrying about meeting a deadline at work may be what keeps you awake. Drinking too much alcohol may disturb your sleep, but worrying about money may be what causes you to drink. So while it is important to ensure that avoidable outside factors do not contribute to sleeplessness, be sure not to ignore the possibility of complex underlying causes for your problem.

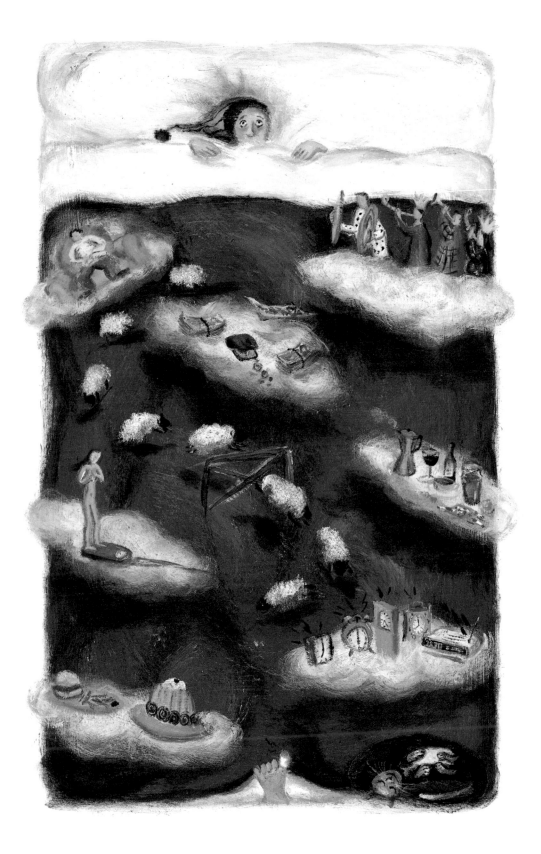

Disruption of the body clock

Modern lifestyles are often governed more by the need to earn a living than the rhythms of nature, and this can take a toll on sleep patterns and, ultimately, health. Twenty-four hour production schedules, world-wide travel, and partying into the early hours of the morning means disturbed biological rhythms and disrupted sleep schedules. Numerous studies have shown that disturbances to the usual sleep routine can have an unhealthy effect on both mind and body.

Shift work

Those who work night shifts are never working in harmony with their body, and rarely feel as good or work as well as they could during the day. Night-shift workers tend to suffer from reduced efficiency, constant tiredness, irritability, and poor decision-making, increasing the risk of industrial accidents and errors of professional judgement. In theory, the circadian rhythm adjusts to a new routine, but in practice shift workers never really adjust. This is partly because on rest days shift workers tend to revert to a normal schedule and daytime *zeitgebers*, particularly sunlight, reset the body clock. In addition, certain body rhythms, particularly fluctuations in body temperature, do not adjust to night work.

Night work also alters sleep patterns. Those who work nights have been shown to sleep longer than those who work normal hours, but for shorter periods at a time, which affects the quality of their sleep. They have less REM sleep than people who sleep at regular times, spend longer in stage one (light) sleep, and wake more frequently. Even those who manage to get enough deep sleep may find it unrefreshing because their hormones are working at cross purposes (*see* p.26). A shift worker who goes into deep sleep at 8am will still produce growth hormone because growth hormone is released during deep sleep, but he or she will also produce the daytime hormones, adrenaline and corticosteroids, because their production

---

Advice for night-shift workers

For those who have to work night shifts there are various ways to reduce sleepiness at work and its ill-effects.

♦ Take a nap before you start your shift.

♦ Take regular exercise.

♦ Do not drink alcohol, especially before going to work.

♦ Consult your doctor about the best time to take any medications.

♦ Work in bright, preferably full-spectrum light.

♦ Improve sleep hygiene as described in Part Three.

is not governed by sleep. This clash of hormones results in inefficient body repair and growth, and unrefreshing sleep.

Jet lag and irregular bedtimes

Jet lag and keeping irregular bedtimes and rising times affect health and vitality levels in a similar way to working shifts. Jet lag in particular can cause various symptoms which result from a disrupted body clock. Daytime sleepiness and being unable to sleep at night, feeling generally unwell with a headache, loss of appetite, irregular bowel movements, and inability to concentrate are the most notable effects. Symptoms tend to be worse when you fly west to east because time shifts ahead while the circadian rhythm lags behind, and they become more severe the more time zones you cross. Quality of sleep is also affected. Instead of having most of your deep sleep at the beginning of the night, it is peppered throughout the sleep period, giving the impression of poorer quality sleep.

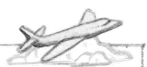

How to combat jet lag

It is possible to relieve the symptoms of jet lag and hasten adjustment by following some basic guidelines when flying across time zones.

♦ Take a night flight if possible, and try to sleep.

♦ Eat only a little light food on the plane.

♦ Avoid alcohol on the flight and drink plenty of water.

♦ Adopt the routine of the new time zone at once.

♦ Try to start the day with some gentle exercise.

♦ Increase your exposure to natural light during the first few days after your flight.

Using naps

Napping has its benefits and its disadvantages (*see also* pp.40-1). The most important disadvantage is that sleeping during the day can mean that you are simply not tired enough to sleep at night. But the judicious use of naps can be beneficial if they help you stay reasonably alert at work and still allow you to sleep at night. In fact many sleep researchers believe that the careful use of napping can strengthen the circadian rhythm and improve mood and concentration.

Concentration naturally dips around eight hours after waking. If you take a short nap of 10 to 15 minutes at about this time it is unlikely to imperil sleep at night, but naps at any other time, particularly 10 to 12 hours after waking, can disturb sleep. If you regularly sleep badly at night, and therefore feel the need to nap the next day, you have probably developed bad sleep habits. To get back to a normal routine, it is important to stay awake during the day. It can take up to ten weeks to restore normal sleep patterns, so be patient.

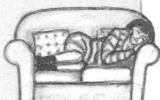

Physical and psychological health

Ill-health, whether it is caused by chronic or serious conditions, injury, or common complaints, is one of the main causes of disrupted sleep. Pain, in particular, makes it difficult to get to sleep, reduces the amount of deep sleep, and often results in broken sleep. Whether the pain is associated with a simple infection or serious illness such as cancer, it disrupts sleep at a time when the body needs it most.

Under- and over-stimulation

People who take little physical exercise during the day may find they are not tired enough to get to sleep at night, and even those who do get to sleep may not be getting the quality of sleep they need. It has been shown that lack of physical activity can seriously affect sleep quality so that you do not function efficiently or wake feeling refreshed. In his book *Insomnia and Other Sleeping Problems,* Dr Peter Lambley uses the term "malsomnia" to describe light, broken sleep with too little deep and REM sleep, characteristic of those who lead an inactive life.

Physical inactivity is not the only type of inactivity that is damaging to sleep. Lack of mental activity, personal motivation, and lack of fulfilment can also contribute to light, broken, and unrefreshing sleep. Malsomnia is believed to be common among people who avoid challenges and whose lives are boring and unfulfilled.

Whereas lack of exercise is ill-advised, too much activity, especially late in the evening, is equally damaging to sleep. Physical exertion releases adrenaline, which paradoxically increases arousal as well as producing tiredness. Mental stimulation late in the evening,

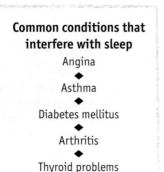

Common conditions that interfere with sleep

Angina

◆

Asthma

◆

Diabetes mellitus

◆

Arthritis

◆

Thyroid problems

ME and fibromyalgia

ME (myalgic encephalomyelitis) is a debilitating condition that causes fatigue, depression, flu-like symptoms, and poor sleep. Fibromyalgia has similar symptoms to ME but is characterized by muscle fatigue and multiple tender points on the body. During sleep sufferers from both conditions produce the alpha-type brain waves associated with relaxed wakefulness instead of theta waves, which normally occur as you fall asleep, or the delta waves of deep sleep. *See* Waking unrested, p.75.

Chemical disrupters of sleep

What you put into your body during the day affects its functioning both throughout the day and during the night. Many substances have the potential to interfere with sleep. To achieve sufficient restful sleep it is important to reduce intake of these chemicals to a minimum.

Caffeine

Caffeine is a stimulant drug found not only in coffee, but also in tea, cocoa, cola drinks, chocolate, and in some prescription and over-the-counter cold and pain- relief preparations. Its adverse effects can last for up to 14 hours. Caffeine-containing drinks give a temporary energy boost because they draw on the body's reserves of energy-giving glycogen and convert it into glucose (sugar). Repeatedly withdrawing from this energy bank means reserves are quickly depleted and you feel constantly tired. However, restorative sleep is also denied you because caffeine stimulates the nervous system and increases adrenaline production, keeping you wide awake and anxious.

Alcohol

Alcohol may send you to sleep quickly, but you are likely to wake in the night owing to a "rebound" effect. Alcohol with caffeine is even more disruptive. Alcohol may initially suppress the stimulating effect of caffeine, but you are likely to wake in early hours of the morning when the effect of the alcohol has worn off.

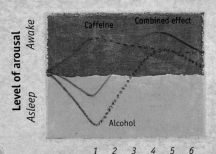

Time after ingestion (hours)

Nicotine

The nicotine in tobacco stimulates the nervous system, raises blood pressure and alters breathing. It also triggers adrenaline release, which inhibits the restorative benefits of sleep. Smokers tend to have lighter, more broken sleep than non-smokers.

Illicit drugs

Many illegal, so-called recreational drugs cause sleep disturbance during use and withdrawal. Disruption to sleep patterns is caused by central nervous system depressants such as cannabis as well as by stimulants such as amphetamines.

Prescribed medications

All drugs have side-effects and a common side-effect of some is sleep disturbance. If you have difficulty sleeping and you are taking any prescription medicine, **do not stop taking the medication**, but discuss the matter with your doctor.

also disturbs sleep, if no "wind-down" time is allowed before bedtime.

Weight loss

People who are slightly heavier than average seem to sleep better than those who are thin. This may be because heavier people are often happier people who have healthier appetites, gain more weight, and sleep better when happy than those who are depressed or anxious, but it is weight rather than body fat that makes the difference. There is also some evidence that heavier people have an ultradian rhythm (*see* p.31) that is longer than average. Longer sleep cycles allow more REM sleep. Losing excess weight may be beneficial for health, but sudden weight loss has been shown to be highly damaging to sleep patterns.

Psychological factors

It has been estimated that 85 to 90 per cent of people with psychological problems, such as anxiety and depression, also have sleep problems. Anxiety causes tension and creates conditions in the body that are opposed to sleep. Anxiety is often a temporary problem caused by exams, a job interview, or any other particularly stressful event and passes when the specific cause has been removed. But the problem sometimes has no obvious cause. Severe and prolonged anxiety, whatever its origin, requires professional treatment.

Sleeping badly is also a classic symptom of depression. Depression seems to disrupt the body clock so that those affected have disturbed sleep or sleep at odd times, sometimes staying awake for most of the night and sleeping during the day. Abnormally, most REM sleep occurs early in the night and most deep sleep later. With antidepressant drugs the sleep pattern can be corrected. Medical treatment for the depressive condition is essential but so, too, is sticking to a rigid sleep routine so that you retrain yourself to go to sleep at night and make yourself stay awake during the day.

Dealing with sleeplessness of emotional origin

♦ Try to put into practice the recommendations in Part Three of this book.

♦ Steer clear of alcohol, which can make symptoms worse and solves nothing.

♦ Get outside and exercise every day.

♦ Telephone a comforting friend or member of the family before you go to bed and talk through anything that is distressing you.

♦ If the problem becomes serious or shows no sign of lifting ask your doctor about getting some psychological help.

External factors

Sleep is disturbed not only by what you put inside your body, but also by what goes on around you. Common sense tells us that noise is not conducive to sound sleep, but susceptibility to it is an individual matter. Sensitivity to noise increases with age and researchers have also found that women are more noise-sensitive than men. Of course, at what stage of sleep the noise occurs also matters. It takes much more to wake us from deep sleep and REM sleep than it does from the light sleep of stages one and two. Not surprisingly, it has been shown that the more tired you are the less likely you are to wake up even with loud noise. Occasional loud noises have been shown to be more disruptive than constant droning, humming, or ticking. The nature of the noise is also important: a mother may sleep through a violent storm, but wakes the instant she hears her baby whimper. Many people woken by noise are kept awake by the anger they feel at having their sleep disturbed.

See Chapter Nine for further advice on making your sleep environment more conducive to sleep.

Temperature changes

You are unlikely to sleep well if you are either too cold or too hot and the quantities of restorative sleep are affected by uncomfortably high or low temperatures. A temperature of around 18°C (65°F) is thought to be ideal for sleep. It has been shown that in temperatures above 24°C (75°F) people wake more frequently, move around more and enjoy less restorative deep and REM sleep. Low temperatures are equally hostile to sleep.

Light

Light and darkness have a special role to play in establishing sleep schedules. These factors also affect the length and quality of our sleep. Exposure to bright light, especially sunlight, in the day promotes restful sleep at night, but at night we need darkness in order to sleep soundly.

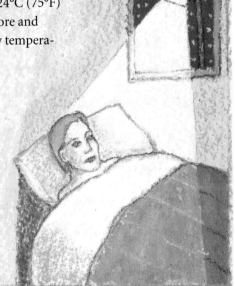

Chapter Six

Sleep disturbance

Up to 65 million Americans and an estimated ten million people in Britain are thought to suffer from poor sleep, and a third of all people who consult a doctor and two thirds of those who see a psychiatrist claim to have unrefreshing and unrestorative sleep. The importance of sleep for physical and mental wellbeing was discussed in Chapter One. Sleep deprivation quickly shows in your face. The skin is a barometer of health and lack of cell renewal means skin cells do not get replaced quickly enough to keep skin plump and glowing. Sags, bags, and dark circles under the eyes are often the first signs of inadequate sleep. Moreover, even one or two sleepless nights can cause enormous anxiety to sufferers. With a little knowledge, however, most sleep disorders can be overcome without professional help. The starting point is an understanding of the nature of your particular problem.

Most people will know what keeps them awake, but it is possible to misdiagnose the cause of the problem. You may wake in the night and find it impossible to get back to sleep because of your partner's snoring, but his or her snoring may not have woken you in the first place. It may have been a bad dream, anxiety, or pain. The questionnaires in the introduction to the book (pp.9-10) are designed to help you analyse the cause of your sleep problem. When you find the cause you can take steps to eradicate the problem or at least limit its effects by making changes to your health and lifestyle, perhaps by reviewing your diet, learning to relax, and following a sleep-inducing bedtime routine. Part Three offers advice on what to do help yourself get the sleep you need.

The American Sleep Disorders Association uses the *yin/yang* symbol to represent the importance of balance between sleeping and waking in maintaining good health.

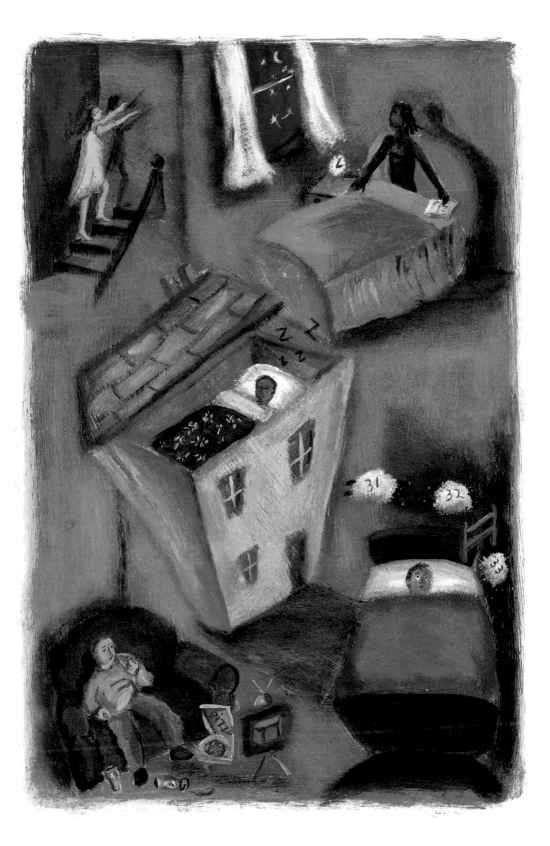

What is insomnia?

Insomnia means inability to sleep. The term can be used to describe difficulty in getting to sleep or staying asleep, as well as a perceived inability to sleep at all. Not all people who sleep little are insomniacs. The difference between short sleepers and insomniacs is that the former need very little sleep to stay healthy and well, while the latter suffer physically and mentally from lack of sleep. Insomnia is not an illness in itself, but a symptom of imbalance in the body and can have many causes.

Transient and short-term insomnia

It is common to be kept awake by nervousness the night before an examination, an important job interview, or one's wedding, and thinking about a sudden piece of exciting news – good or bad – can similarly make sleep hard to achieve. Anxiety excites the nervous system and keeps the brain awake and agitated (*see* facing page). Transient insomnia can be brought on not only by stress, but also by minor health problems such as coughs and colds, by disruption to the body clock as in jet lag, and external disturbances such as noise. The cause of this type of sleep difficulty is usually obvious, and the problem disappears when the cause is eliminated. Short-term insomnia is of longer duration, and can last for two to three weeks. It is often the result of emotional upheaval such as divorce, bereavement, pain, or illness.

Where short-term insomnia is the result of an emotional problem, counselling, or even talking things through with a friend, can help. Hypnotherapy can also be beneficial in clearing out repressed emotions, and many other complementary therapies such as homeopathy, aromatherapy, and acupuncture that work to restore emotional as well as physical health can also help to get you through these difficult periods (*see* Part Four). For some people sleeping pills can be invaluable for promoting sleep during short periods of severe distress or pain (*see* Chapter Eleven).

Chronic insomnia

Sleeping difficulties that persist over a longer period –
chronic insomnia – may also be caused by psychological,
environmental, or physiological problems. Sometimes a
traumatic event such as an accident, death in the family,
or divorce can trigger the problem, which may then
become ingrained, particularly if you become reliant
on sleeping pills. Long-term lifestyle or environmental
factors such as alcohol dependency or job-related stress
may also lead to chronic insomnia. Certain drugs and
long-term medical conditions also have their part to play
in the development of long-standing sleeping problems.

Difficulty getting to sleep

Habitual sleeplessness does not affect everyone in the
same way and often the pattern of sleeplessness can give
clues to its causes. Both short-term and chronic insomnia
can be divided into several types. Almost half of all those
with sleeping difficulties have a problem getting to sleep.
Many people who claim to have difficulty falling asleep,

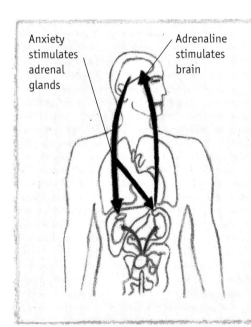

Anxiety
stimulates
adrenal
glands

Adrenaline
stimulates
brain

**Hormone activity and
wakefulness**

Anxiety produces the same
physiological effects as
confrontation with danger.
The brain sends messages to
the adrenal glands to produce
adrenaline, which in turn
heightens alertness. People
who are kept awake by anxiety
often find that even when
they do go to sleep, they wake
unrefreshed. This is because
the high levels of adrenaline
block the restorative action
of growth hormone.

when woken from light (stage one and two) sleep do not feel they have been asleep at all, indicating that their experience of sleep is rather different from so-called "normal" sleepers. This perception that they cannot sleep at all seems to adds to the insomniac's anxiety and makes the problem worse.

If you find yourself lying in bed trying to get to sleep for more than 30 minutes, try not to get worked up about it. Remember, your ultradian rhythm (*see* p.31) dictates that within the space of 90 to 100 minutes you will experience a period of drowsiness, during which you can fall asleep quite easily. Instead of tossing and turning in bed get up, go into another room, and do something relaxing or boring for a while. Have a cup of herb tea if you like, but not a caffeine-containing drink. When you feel sleepy go back to bed and try again.

Anxiety, anger, and stress are among the most common causes of wakefulness. Stress-management and relaxation techniques can be beneficial in controlling day-to-day anxiety (*see also* Part Three). People who suffer from constant or recurrent anxiety should seek medical help. Successful treatment of the underlying cause of anxiety often clears up the sleep problem without the need for further action.

In traditional Chinese medicine, problems with falling asleep usually indicate blood deficiency, which can be caused by worry and anxiety or too little protein in the diet. Other symptoms of blood deficiency include pins and needles, cramps caused by poor circulation, poor concentration, and a poor memory. The latter two are also recognized by orthodox western medicine as classic symptoms of lack of sleep.

Night waking

Because we move through cycles of light, deep, and REM sleep, we all dip in and out of periods of wakefulness during sleep. These usually occur after REM sleep, but we do not remember them because they are so brief. Some

Involuntary movements

Some people wake frequently during the night with involuntary jerks of the legs – a condition known as restless legs. Iron deficiency and too much tea, which contains caffeine and hinders iron absorption in the body, have been suggested as triggers. Calcium and other vitamin and mineral deficiencies have also been blamed. It may also be related to poor circulation. Drug treatment is not always effective. The alternatives include taking more exercise, and vitamin and mineral supplementation. Ginkgo biloba may also be helpful.

people, however, can lie awake for what seems like hours. Depression, anxiety, pain, respiratory illness, alcohol, caffeine, drug abuse, and the frequent need to go to the toilet can all contribute to such extended night wakings.

In traditional Chinese medicine waking frequently is due to a deficiency of *yin* energy, which can be caused by overwork, stress, emotional strain, and poor diet. Chinese medical practitioners see *yin* deficiency as a common cause of insomnia in the elderly. *Yin* is described as cold and wet. Symptoms of deficiency can include feeling hot, hot flushes, anger, constipation, and restlessness, all of which are known to interfere with sleep quality.

Early waking

The tendency to wake early increases with age. It is well-established that sleep gets lighter as we get older and for many people this means waking as soon as it starts to get light or when it begins to get noisy outside. You can take measures to darken your room or block out external noise (*see* Chapter Nine), but you also need to be realistic about your sleep needs and accept that it is natural to wake early as you get older rather than trying to fight it.

Ayurvedic medicine also views lighter, shorter periods of sleep as a natural development. According to this ancient system, different ages of life, like every other aspect of nature, are dominated by different *doshas* (*see* p.19). After the age of 40, active *vata* energy increases and this means sleep is more easily disturbed, particularly in the early hours of the morning (2am to 4am). In people who already have an imbalance in *vata* energy, this naturally light sleep can progress to insomnia.

Western psychiatrists see early waking as a classic sign of endogenous depression (feelings of sadness that are not linked to any outside event). Early waking on its own does not signify depression, but it may be a possibility if combined with additional symptoms such as apathy, loss of appetite and sex drive, unexplained muscular aches, and possibly morbid thoughts. (*See also* p.68.)

Waking unrested
A small number of people suffer from what is known as alpha-delta sleep during which the brain wave patterns of wakefulness continue through deep sleep. Such people get very little restorative deep sleep. They can sleep for six to eight hours yet wake up and claim they have not slept at all. Their sleep is unrefreshing and sufferers get up feeling as tired as when they went to bed.

Snoring and sleep apnoea

Snoring is often considered more of a problem for a sleep partner than for the snorer him- or herself. But it can disrupt the sleep of both partners and has even been known to disturb sleepers in the next room. Between a third and a half of all adults snore. Men seem to make the noisiest bed partners, although a number of women are affected after the menopause.

What causes snoring?

Snoring is caused by an obstruction in the upper airways – either in the nose or throat. When we are asleep the muscles of the upper neck and inside the throat are relaxed, and lack of support from weak or flabby throat muscles means that the soft palate (the tissues at the back of the throat) easily vibrates with each inhaled breath. These vibrations cause characteristic snoring sounds.

As we get older, the throat muscles get weaker, making snoring more likely. Being overweight is also a contributory factor. Fat affects the functioning of all the muscles in the body including those in the throat. A blocked nose from a cold or allergy can cause temporary snoring, as can nasal polyps and enlarged adenoids or tonsils. Problems such as goitre and an overactive thyroid gland are also possible risk factors. Children who snore usually have enlarged tonsils or adenoid problems. In adults heavy drinking, consumption of sleeping pills, smoking, and sleeping on your back all increase the likelihood of snoring.

Effects on health and wellbeing

People who snore may not even know that they do it and may happily sleep through the night without waking. However, many others who snore have fragmented sleep that leaves them tired, irritable, and sleepy the following day. Nevertheless, for most people simple snoring is not a serious health risk, although it may indicate health and lifestyle problems that should be rectified. A more severe problem, related to snoring, is known as sleep apnoea.

What happens when we snore

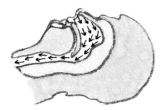

During sleep the muscles that control the tongue and soft palate should hold the airway open.

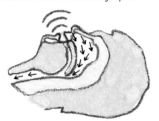

If the muscles become slack, the airway is narrowed, which causes snoring and breathing difficulties.

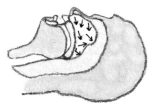

In some cases the airway is periodically completely blocked, preventing breathing. This is obstructive sleep apnoea.

Sleep apnoea

The condition is characterized by loud snoring and frequent choking attacks during the night. The choking occurs because the soft palate is sucked closed when the sleeper breathes in, blocking the airways and temporarily stopping breathing causing the sleeper to choke and wake up gasping for breath. These choking episodes can last from 10 to 90 seconds and may, in severe cases, occur up to 1,000 times a night. The causes of sleep apnoea are similar to those of snoring.

These frequent wakenings lead to marked daytime sleepiness, which is a major feature of the condition. In extreme cases the sleepiness can be so severe that it prevents sufferers from working or driving. Some people who have tried to carry on with everyday tasks have caused serious and often fatal accidents at home, work, or on the road. American researchers estimate that 20 per cent of people with sleep apnoea have had car accidents as a result of falling asleep at the wheel.

The risks of sleep apnoea

The dangers associated with daytime sleepiness are not the only cause for concern with sleep apnoea. When breathing is obstructed during light or deep sleep the lack of oxygen prompts the brain to send emergency signals to the muscles to move. But the problem is usually at its worst during REM sleep and it is here that it is also most dangerous. The muscular paralysis that occurs during REM sleep means the body takes longer to respond to the fact that the brain is getting less oxygen. Thankfully, such serious sleep apnoea is rare, affecting only one to two per cent of the population.

Sleep apnoea sufferers tend to be moody, constantly tired and have little interest in sex. They have very little REM sleep and, in severe cases, virtually no deep sleep. Lack of REM sleep combined with the breathing problems that result in reduced oxygen getting to the brain may explain why those with sleep apnoea frequently develop memory and intellect problems.

High blood pressure, heart disease, and increased risk of stroke are all associated with sleep apnoea. In America every year 2,000 to 3,000 sleep apnoea sufferers die as a result of night-time heart attacks. For asthmatics and people with other respiratory diseases the risks of nightly breathing difficulties are obvious.

Ways to reduce snoring

There is general agreement among professionals that drugs have no part to play in the treatment of snoring and sleep apnoea. Self-help measures and numerous devices appear to be more successful. Snoring, like insomnia, is a symptom rather than a disease. Exercising, losing weight, drinking less alcohol, not smoking, and staying off sedative drugs are the first, commonsense steps for better health and less snoring.

Throat exercises
In her book *The Natural Way to Stop Snoring*, Dr Elizabeth Scott maintains that professional singers rarely snore because they give their throat muscles a regular workout. Dr Scott advises losing weight, doing deep breathing and yawning exercises, clearing your nasal passages, smiling, gargling, stretching your tongue, and singing. You might find you enjoy the exercises and apart from reduced snoring, singing is a great stress buster.

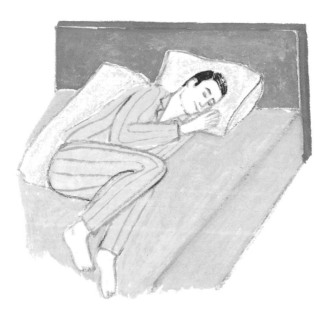

Sleeping on your side

Sleeping on your side or stomach rather than your back can help to minimize snoring. When you lie on your back your tongue is more likely to slide back towards your throat and block the air flow. The traditional advice to stop you rolling back on to your back is to sew a tennis ball into the back of your pyjamas. The more favoured alternative is to put pillows behind you.

Anti-snoring treatments

Anti-snoring devices work to some degree to reduce the noise of snoring, and counter the health risks of sleep apnoea, but they do not address the cause. Nasal clips or strips favoured by sportsmen and women who want to improve their oxygen intake can also help with snoring in some cases. These clips, available from pharmacies, are fixed to the outside of the nose to open the nostrils and improve breathing. A more complicated but extremely effective alternative is the CPAP (continuous positive airway pressure) device. This consists of a nasal mask that is strapped onto the face, to deliver air at a slightly higher pressure than normal and so keep the airways open. Although it may seem unnatural to wear this bizarre-looking device, it oftens bring about dramatic improvements for sleep apnoea patients.

There is also an anti-snoring operation, known as uvulopalatopharyngoplasty. The surgeon cauterizes the soft palate to make it more rigid and less likely to flap. It is a drastic measure that does not always work, but it can produce some improvement and may be valuable to the most high-risk apnoea patients. The risk for those for whom surgery does not work is that it may also make CPAP ineffective because of damage to the soft palate. Other operations are still experimental, although some doctors are quieting snorers with a laser surgery technique, called laser assisted uvulopalatoplasty. It is not usually suitable for the obese or those whose snoring is caused by problems other than a flabby soft palate.

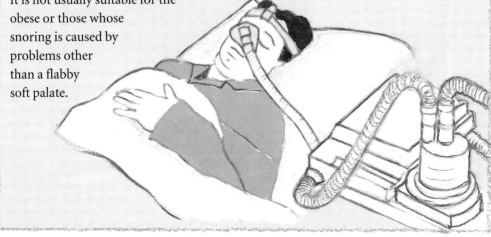

Sleep-walking and parasomnias

Sleep-walking (somnambulism) is one of a group of sleep disturbances known collectively as parasomnias. This term is used to cover several undesirable physical phenomena that occur during sleep. Bedwetting, night terrors, and teeth grinding, for example, are other forms of parasomnia. About 15 per cent of people sleep-walk at some time in their lives. The phemonomen is most common in children (For more information, *see* Chapter Seven). Most adults who sleep-walk tend to do so during periods of anxiety or stress or because they keep irregular sleep schedules. Shiftworkers or people who go without sleep for long periods are more likely to sleep-walk, possibly because they get more deep sleep than people who keep regular hours. Consumption of alcohol, which confuses the sleep/wake mechanism, sleep apnoea, and conditions such as migraine and epileptic fits are also associated with sleep-walking.

Adults who have a tendency to sleep-walk should stick to regular bedtimes, avoid getting too tired, and steer clear of shift work, if possible. Stress and anxiety can be a contributory factor so try some form of stress management or a relaxation technique to help you wind down in the evening. If the problem may be related to some more deep-rooted anxiety or personality problem counselling may help. Many of the safety suggestions for child sleep-walkers (*see* p.87) are also applicable to adults.

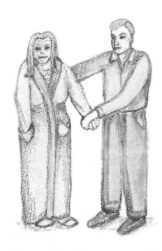

What to do when someone is night-wandering

If you find someone sleep-walking or night-wandering, gently steer him or her back to bed, reassure them that everything is all right, and switch off the light. Try to avoid a confrontation even if this means accompanying them on a short walk before returning to bed.

Night-wandering

Elderly people, especially those with Alzheimer's disease or other forms of dementia, are prone to night-wandering. Night-wandering is not sleep-walking. Those affected are awake, it is simply that their short-term memory is impaired and they become confused about whether it is night or day. Sometimes a change of environment can lead to disorientation. A new house, or even a change of room, can be confusing. Excess energy is another possible cause of night-wandering. Exercise is important for sound sleep whatever your age. Too often elderly people do not get physically tired during the day. Try to make sure that any elderly person in your care gets some gentle exercise outdoors each day. Social interaction is also important for ensuring satisfyingly stimulating days.

Attention should be given to the same sleep hygiene rules outlined in Part Three. Many elderly people go to bed too early, perhaps because they are bored, cold, or because they have always gone to bed early. It helps to make a clear distinction between night and day by keeping the house bright during the daytime and turning off all lights at night, although a gentle night light can be reassuring. Try to avoid confusion by keeping familiar objects and furniture in their usual place, so that the person does not become disorientated. If someone in your care continues to wander, make sure their environment is as safe as possible by locking windows and outside doors.

Bruxism

Bruxism, or teeth grinding, occurs mainly during stages one and two of sleep. In the long term, bruxism can cause damage to the teeth by wearing away the enamel and stressing the joints of the jaw. However, the more immediate effect is waking up to facial pain and earache and, in some cases, recurrent headaches. The cause is unclear, although anxiety seems to be a primary cause. There is no specific medical treatment for bruxism, but children and people for whom bruxism causes regular pain and tooth damage can wear a rubber mouth or bite guard that protects the teeth.

Sleep paralysis

Sleep paralysis occurs when you are waking from a dream. Your body is still asleep and completely immobile. The feelings soon disappear, but the experience can be frightening.

Narcolepsy

Narcolepsy is an extremely rare incurable condition that is mainly genetically determined. It is estimated that only 0.15 per cent of the population suffer from this condition. It is characterized by excessive daytime sleepiness and instant paralysis similar to that which takes place during REM sleep. Sufferers can fall asleep at any time, even while driving short distances and while having sex, when surging adrenaline levels ought to keep them awake. The condition seems to be at its worst around the age of 20. The hazards of narcolepsy are obvious. It is dangerous to drive or operate machinery, your work and personal relationships suffer. Doctors sometimes prescribe amphetamines which can help some people to stay alert during the day.

Chapter Seven

Childhood sleep problems

Children's health and development depends on balance, which among other things includes a balance between rest and activity and waking and sleeping. Good quality sleep is essential to enable a child to work, play, and absorb the enormous amount of information they need to grow into competent adults. Without good sleep children can lose their natural energy and alertness and become overtired, irritable, apathetic, and moody. Children have a tremendous amount of energy that needs to be directed into physical activities so that they happily exhaust themselves during the day and get the sleep they need at night. Sleeping may be as natural as breathing, but good sleep habits need to be learned. Some child care experts insist that it is as much a parent's responsibility to ensure that their children get the sleep they need as it is to ensure they eat a healthy diet.

How much sleep do children need?

Babies have no idea of time. They go to sleep when they are tired, not because it is bedtime. Like older people, their body rhythms respond to light and dark, but their ultradian rhythms are shorter so they tend to wake much more frequently demanding food and attention. As they grow their sleep patterns become more like those of adults. Given the chance, however, babies and young children will still wake up in the night, especially if they get rewarded with kisses and cuddles.

Most sleep experts agree that serious sleep deprivation can affect a child's development, but opinions vary about

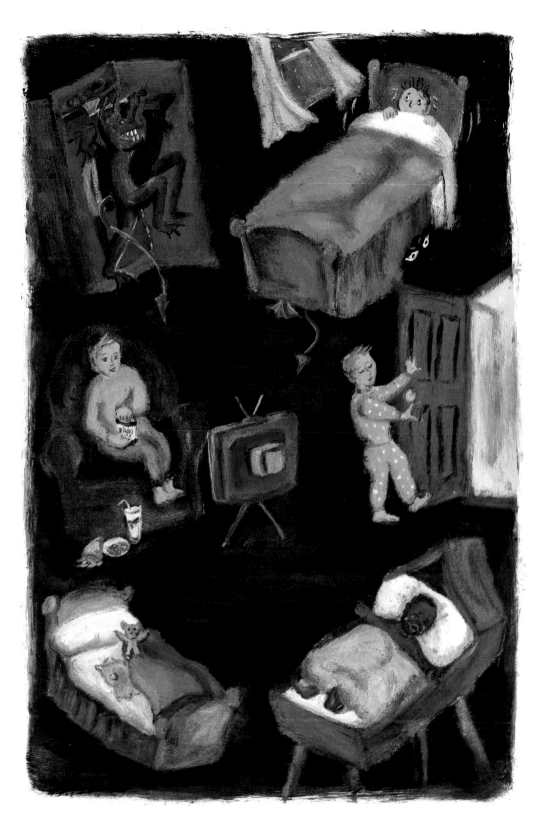

the prevalence of sleep deprivation among children. Some babies seem to thrive on little sleep and those who do tend to grow up needing less sleep than average. Every child is an individual and the average sleep patterns described here should be used as a guide only.

Realistic expectations

The most important starting point is to assess if your expectations are realistic. Most parents expect to have sleepless nights, but some are more tolerant than others. Researchers who polled mothers to find out if they believed their babies had a sleep problem found that parental tolerance was an important benchmark in assessing the quality of a child's sleep. Although some children do have obvious sleep problems, others simply do not measure up to their parents' expectations of what is "normal" for a child of their age. A child who doesn't sleep as much as his or her parents think appropriate may have a physical, psychological, or emotional problem, or it

Newborn to 12 weeks

Newborn babies can sleep for 16 hours out of 24. Babies need frequent brief periods of sleep, alternating with periods of wakefulness that allow for frequent feeds. It is normal for an infant to have erratic sleep patterns. As the child settles down his or her sleep will gradually become more regular.

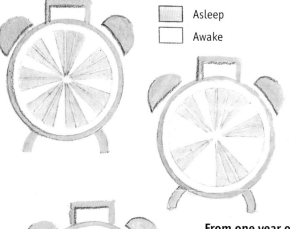

Asleep

Awake

12 weeks to one year

As they get older, children have less frequent but more prolonged sleeps. By the age of three months it has been estimated that 70 per cent of babies have an undisturbed night's sleep. A long period of sleep at night is usually supplemented by one or more periods of daytime sleep.

From one year onward

At this age children spend the night moving between light sleep and REM sleep. These phases are punctuated by periods of arousal when the child wakes up, changes position, or seems half asleep. Often they simply go back to sleep, but sometimes the period of arousal becomes extended. Children usually continue to need a daytime nap until around the age of three.

could simply be that the child is not tired or has a vested interest in staying awake.

Occasionally illness or anxiety can keep a child awake. Children are very sensitive to arguments between their parents and major life crises such as separation or divorce can make them feel vulnerable, anxious, and restless. These are special situations that call for love, support, and reassurance in every area of the child's life. The sleeping problem should resolve once the underlying problem has been dealt with.

If you can identify recognizable sleep disturbances such as the common ones detailed below there are certain steps you can take to correct them. If you believe your child has a serious sleep problem, contact your family doctor, who may be able to refer you to a specialist for help.

Bad sleep habits

If you have a healthy, happy child who refuses to go to sleep every night, the cause may be the habits you are teaching your child. Children need comfort, reassurance, and love, but they also need and respond to routine. They thrive on stability and discipline, and they benefit from knowing that there is a right time and place for every-thing, including going to sleep. It is important to establish a sensible bedtime routine that gives your child time to wind down for bed and ensures he or she gets enough sleep (*see* pp.90-1).

Waking in the night

Depending on their age and circumstances children can wake for all sorts of reasons. Young babies can be hungry, colicky, unwell, cold, or hot, and older children can be lonely, frightened, or stressed by something that has hap-pened at home, nursery, or school. Night terrors (p.88) can also appear to disturb sleep although they do not actually wake the child. Between 6 and 18 months some children start to wake frequently during the night. It often starts when illness or teething wakes the child and he or

Evening colic
Many babies between the ages of two weeks and three months are kept awake by evening (or three-month) colic. Nobody is sure why some babies get colic; it may be wind, hunger, overfeed-ing, indigestion, or tension. Babies are very sensitive to the moods of those around them and they can pick up on feelings of tension.

Holding and comforting the baby is a natural response. Some parents manage the problem with over-the-counter prepara-tions such as gripe water, or natural alternatives. Dietary changes by mothers who are breast-feeding may help.

Breaking the crying habit

There is no one right way to deal with crying, sleepless babies. Some experts advise putting your baby to bed and leaving him or her to cry him- or herself to sleep. Other people believe you should never leave a child to cry because they become withdrawn and emotionally scarred by the neglect, although there has been no evidence to suggest that this is true. Two methods are described here. Parents must decide for themselves which approach is more suitable for them.

Leaving your child to cry

♦ Put your child to bed, say goodnight and leave the room.

♦ If your child cries, check that he or she is not wet, soiled, sick, or in pain or danger.

♦ When he or she is settled leave the room.

♦ If your child starts to cry again, leave him or her to cry him- or herself to sleep.

♦ If your child wakes later in the night repeat the procedure. The hope is that each time your child wakes the crying will last for a shorter time.

Advantages

♦ Those who follow the plan correctly and do not give in to the crying usually see results within a week.

♦ The child learns to become an independent sleeper, so you can put him or her to bed in the knowledge that he or she will fall asleep.

Disadvantages

♦ You need to be very patient and tolerant. Parents who cannot bear to hear their child cry are unlikely to endure several days of the sort of trauma that is necessary for success.

♦ Several nights of noise, guilt, and anxiety for you.

♦ It is not suitable for older children who can get out of bed and go to you for comfort.

The softly softly method

♦ Put your child to bed as normal and decide that if he or she does not sleep or wakes during the night you will allow crying to continue for a certain time before you intervene.

♦ When you go to your child, give comfort for only one or two minutes and then leave. Don't stay until he or she stops crying or goes to sleep.

♦ Next time let him or her cry a little longer before intervening, and the time after that a little longer still. Continue like this through-out the night and on successive nights.

Advantages

♦ Frequent checks relieve parental anxiety and stops you imagining what could be wrong with your baby.

♦ The child does not feel deserted and you feel less guilty about letting him or her cry.

Disadvantages

♦ Only suitable after the age of about six months.

♦ Can take quite a long time for the child to achieve an uninterrupted night's sleep

♦ It is hard to be sufficiently patient or disciplined to see the plan through.

♦ Your brief visits may distress the child, having the opposite effect from that intended.

she gets used to getting nightly attention. To break this sort of habit, try following the advice on the facing page.

Nevertheless, a child who wakes several times during the night in a state of distress needs to be comforted. Go to the child and soothe him or her, say gently that you are there and everything is all right, but try not to take the child out of bed or turn on the light. Reassure the child that it is safe to go back to sleep and leave the room.

Sleep-walking

Sleep-walking most often occurs during deep sleep in the first third of the night. This extra allocation of deep sleep may explain why sleep-walking is more common in children. Most children who sleep-walk start before the age of ten. More boys than girls are affected, and there is evidence that sleep-walking runs in families. In affected children the sleep and waking mechanisms are confused so that the sleep-walker can carry out everyday activities such as dressing and walking perfectly well, but without being aware of what they are doing. Sleep-walks can last from a few minutes to an hour and when they wake up the sleep-walker rarely remembers what they were doing or why they got out of bed. Those who walk in their sleep also tend to talk in their sleep. As with adults, episodes of sleep-walking in children can be related to periods of anxiety or stress. Some scientists claim that sleep-walking can be caused by geopathic stress (*see* Chapter Nine).

There is little you can do to prevent sleep-walking and in time most children simply grow out of the habit. However, it is important to make the sleep environment of a child who sleep-walks as safe as possible. Lock doors and windows and put a stairgate at the top of the stairs. Few sleep-walkers perform any daring or unusual manoeuvres and most are adept at negotiating obstacles or perilous routes. However, the child can become confused and disorientated so it is important to remove all possible risks. If you encounter your child while he or she is sleep-walking, gently steer him or her back to bed.

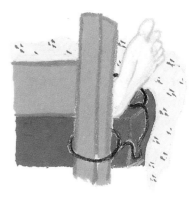

Keeping your child safe
If you are particularly concerned you could also tie the child to the bed. This does not mean strapping them in so that they cannot move, but a fairly long piece of string tied loosely around the ankle and fastened to the bed post ensures that they don't wander off too far.

Nightmares

Nearly half of all children start to have nightmares between the ages of three and six. It is not clear why children have these disturbing experiences. Some psychologists suggest that six-year-olds are at an age where they are struggling to understand the concept of death and sleep. During sleep those morbid fears come to the surface in the form of nightmares. Of course children also worry about family tensions, school work, and bullying. They also watch television and videos, read books, play games, and meet people who frighten them. Suppressed fears can find an outlet in dreams.

Children often remember their dreams and you can find out quite a lot about what worries your child by asking him or her to tell you what he or she remembers about the bad dream. It is important to give children the support to do this and not force them to talk about things they would rather forget. Tell them it was only a dream and that dreams cannot harm us. (*See also* p.58.)

Night terrors

Night terrors are less common than nightmares, but are also a standard part of childhood sleep experiences, especially between the ages of three and six. Night terrors differ from nightmares in several ways. They occur during the first four hours of sleep rather than during the middle to latter part of the night. They can last from ten minutes to an hour. The child sits up screaming with eyes wide open, disorientated, and probably totally unaware of your presence. There is no evidence to suggest that children are adversely affected by these terrifying episodes; most don't even remember what it was that terrified them, and with a little reassurance they settle back to sleep. There's little you can do for a child experiencing night terrors. Hold the child if he or she lets you, but you are just as likely to be pushed away. Don't try to wake your child, as the likelihood is that you would succeed only in confusing and frightening him or her. All you can do to prevent further

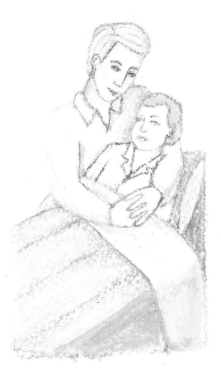

Comforting after a nightmare
A child who has had a nightmare needs to be allowed to describe the dream if he or she wants to. Comfort and reassure the child, that the bad dream was not real.

attacks is to help your child get as much rest as possible as terrors are less likely to occur in children who have had enough sleep.

Bedwetting

Bedwetting, or enuresis, is more common in boys than in girls and, like the other parasomnias, tends to run in families. Some children continue to wet the bed until adolescence. Bedwetting is a sensitive subject and the older the child gets the more sensitive about it they become. Encourage your child to go to the toilet before bedtime, avoid bedtime drinks, but do not withhold drinks if your child is thirsty. You could also try some of the natural remedies described in Part Four. Offer praise after a dry night, but don't punish or blame him or her when "accidents" occur. Making a child feel ashamed or anxious will only make the problem worse.

Bedwetting is rarely caused by physical illness – where it is, there are usually daytime symptoms as well. Most often it is a symptom of psychological distress. The arrival of a new baby, a change of school, or parental separation can trigger bedwetting in children who were previously dry.

Bedwetting when previously dry
If an older child suddenly starts to wet the bed, when this has not been a problem previously, consult your doctor as there is a chance that the cause could be a minor urinary-tract infection.

In most cases of bedwetting, patience and understanding are all that is needed to help the child overcome the problem. However, if the problem is causing severe distress, it is worthwhile seeking professional help. In America, experts in sleep disorders have had some success in programmes in which the child learns improved bladder control. Not all children respond to this sort of training. Some parents find it helps to use a buzzer and pad device. The pad is placed under the child's sheet and the electrical buzzer goes off when the sheet gets wet. The child becomes conditioned into waking and going to the toilet when he or she needs to empty his bladder. This is quite safe and has a good record of success. Some children who wet the bed are prescribed imipramine, a drug more commonly used to treat depression in adults. One of its side-effects is improved bladder control.

Establishing a bedtime routine

Most children feel secure with a regular daily routine that provides a framework for each day's exciting, unpredictable, and occasionally upsetting events. A child who does not feel secure during the day is likely to have a special need for security at night. It is therefore helpful to provide a time at the end of the day when the pleasant rituals of bedtime can help a child put aside any worries, and this may help to prevent night-time disturbances. Even if your child does not have a sleeping problem, it is worthwhile establishing a pleasant bedtime routine, as it is easier to maintain one than to establish a new pre-sleep ritual if sleeping problems arise in the future.

Massage

If you have a restless baby, treat him or her to a massage. Gentle stroking is relaxing for both of you, and can make your baby feel loved and secure.

Bathtime

Most young children love a leisurely bathtime, which provides the opportunity for water play and may be one of the few times when he or she has your undivided atten-tion. Try adding a drop of lavender or chamomile essential oil to the bath water to enhance the relaxation benefits.

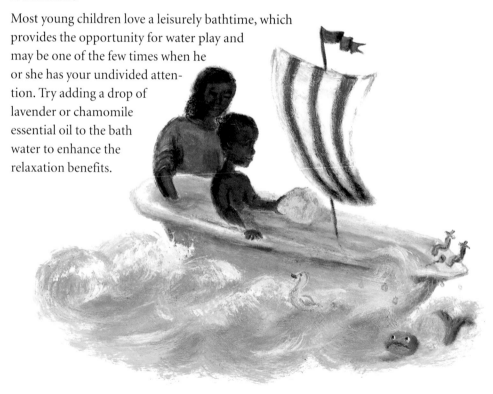

Providing comfort

Bedtimes are important times for giving and receiving affection. A goodnight kiss and cuddle, and a chat about anything that may be troubling your child, is a good way of giving him or her a sense of emotional security before going to sleep.

Keeping to a regular bedtime

For a routine to work it needs to be regular, and a consistent bedtime is an important element in this. Decide on a bedtime for your child and stick to it whenever possible. Changing from night to night or from week to week is unsettling and is likely to prevent him or her developing a regular sleep pattern.

Story time

For many children bedtime story-reading is the most enjoyable part of the evening routine. The expectation of this part of the ritual often has children happily rushing into bed.

Delaying tactics

Be firm about how many stories you are prepared to read. Some children will delay going to sleep by repeatedly asking for more stories. Try agreeing which stories you are going to read before you start.

Points to remember
♦ Plan a routine that suits your family's needs.
♦ Never send a child to bed as a punishment.
♦ Avoid boisterous play before bedtime.

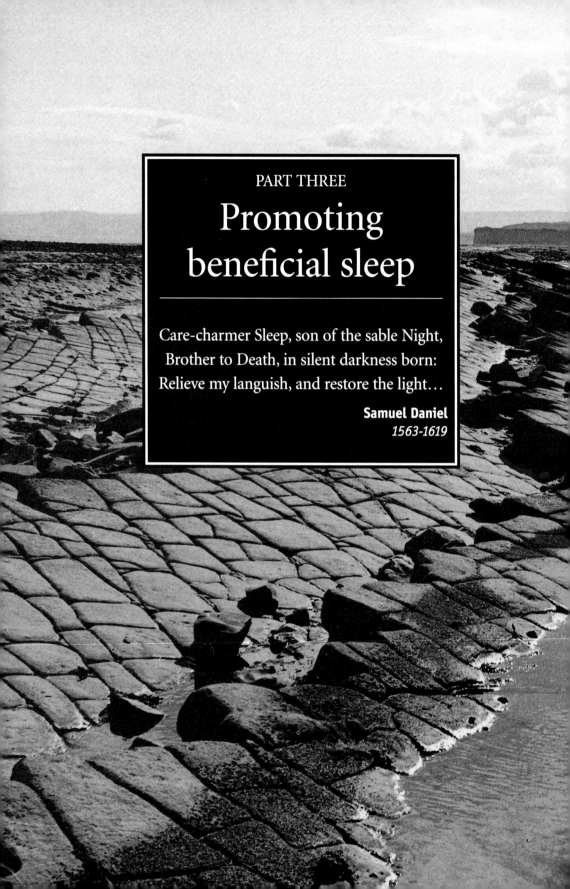

PART THREE

Promoting beneficial sleep

Care-charmer Sleep, son of the sable Night,
Brother to Death, in silent darkness born:
Relieve my languish, and restore the light…

Samuel Daniel
1563-1619

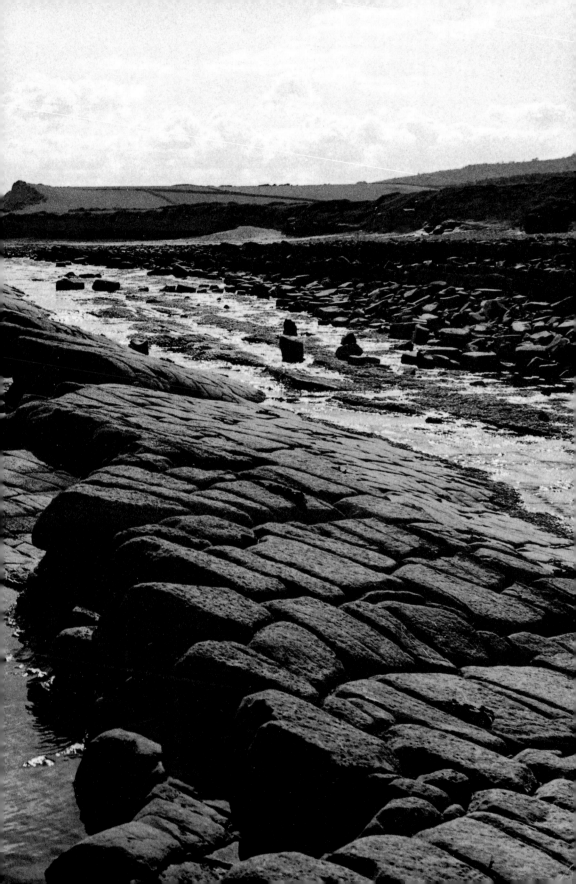

Chapter Eight

Your sleep-friendly day

"In ancient times people who understood the Tao patterned their lives according to yin and yang. And so they lived in harmony. There was temperance in eating and drinking. Their hours of rising and retiring were regular, and their lives were not disorderly and wild. By these means the ancients kept their bodies united with their souls, so as to fulfil their allotted span completely, measuring unto 100 years and more before they passed away."

The Yellow Emperor's Classic
of Internal Medicine
200 BC

For anyone concerned with getting a better night's sleep, paying attention to how you live your life during the day is as important as the strategies you adopt immediately before bedtime. Even chronic insomnia can improve if you make general improvements to health and fitness. A better diet, a more active day, and paying more attention to your emotional health can put your body and mind back in balance so you naturally get the sleep you need. Chapter Five outlined some of the main factors that can interfere with sleep. For a sleep-friendly day, it is important to eliminate or reduce the impact of these factors in your life.

This chapter contains positive advice about eating, sleeping, and living well. It does not take account of individual dietary problems, such as food allergies, or illnesses that make exercise difficult. You probably know better than anyone what you can and cannot do, eat, or achieve. You alone know what you are prepared to do for the sake of your health and happiness. However, if you have a chronic or serious illness, disability, or special dietary needs, it would be advisable to consult your doctor or other health professional before making dramatic changes in your life.

Make an early start

If you act on only one piece of advice in this book make sure it is this: start your sleep-friendly day early. If you want to sleep at night, get up early in the morning. Not just on an occasional morning, but every morning,

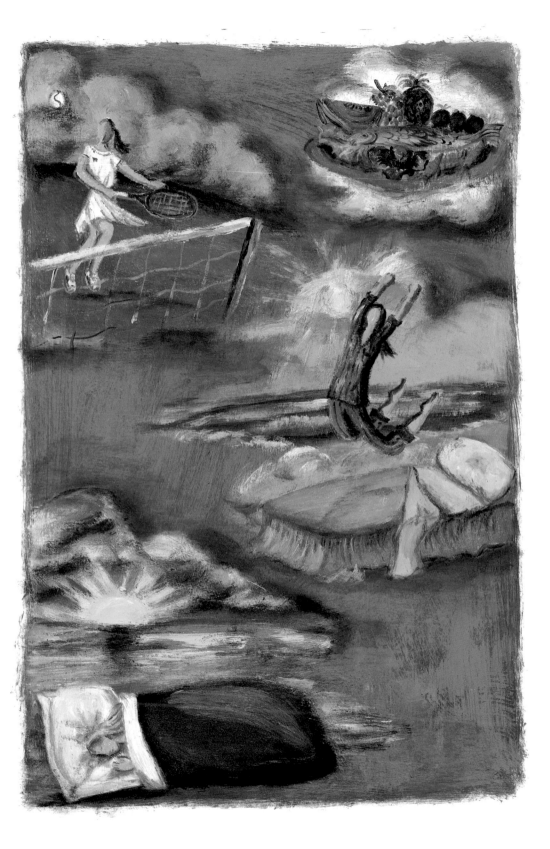

including weekends. Regularity is important in keeping body rhythms constant. Our bodies are programmed to get up early. As described in Chapter One, levels of the wake-up hormones adrenaline and corticosteroids rise in the early morning, acting as a sort of wake-up tonic.

Sleeping in until mid morning means you are not ready to go to sleep until well after midnight, by which time you begin to lose out on sleep's healing benefits. There are also other benefits to getting up early. Talk to early risers and

Light therapy

People who find it difficult to get up early may benefit from light therapy. Special lights designed to simulate full-spectrum daylight are used to stimulate the pineal gland, which regulates body rhythms through the production of hormones serotonin and melatonin (see also p.27). Exposure to bright light in the morning boosts production of serotonin and encourages your body to use up more energy early in the day so that you are ready for bed earlier at night.

It can help to put a lamp on a timer switch in your bedroom. When the lamp switches on, the light should wake you up. Regular use of a full-spectrum light can help you feel more energetic and happier, especially in the winter.

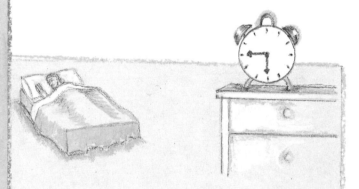

Reinforce your internal body clock

Your body and mind thrive on the discipline of regular cycles of activity and rest. Experiment with how much sleep you need; it may be more or less than the seven to eight hour average. Also decide on the best time for you to go to bed and get up – and stick to it. You can be reasonably flexible about when you can go to bed, but try to make it before midnight.

If your internal body clock is disrupted by years of irregular habits or has recently been upset by jet lag, for example, you will need to restore your body rhythms. The best way to do this is to force yourself to get up early in the morning, even if you are still tired, so that you are ready to go to bed much earlier at night. Invest in an alarm clock that is loud enough to wake you and place it far enough out of reach to make you get out of bed to switch it off. If you set it for the same time every morning it will help to reset your internal clock. It also helps if the room is light when you wake up; so if you have heavy curtains on your windows, put a bright light on a timer switch, again well away from the bed, so that the light will help to wake you up and prevent you from going back to sleep. After a few weeks you may find your body has become so thoroughly re-educated that you wake before the alarm goes off.

they will nearly always tell you that early morning is the best part of the day. There is stillness about early morning that vanishes when the rest of the world comes alive. It provides a period of calm in which to plan the day ahead, go for a walk, swim, meditate, or practise yoga. For many people it is also the most creative time of the day, ideas come more easily and problems seem easier to solve.

Early rising is in keeping with the philosophy of Ayurveda. *Vata*, the *dosha* concerned with movement and activity is predominant in early morning. Anyone who has sleeping problems should be sure to get up in *vata* time – ideally around 6am. According to Ayurveda, not working in harmony with the *doshas* causes chaotic sleep patterns.

Early to bed

Make your lights-out time earlier rather than later. People who go to bed after midnight and get up late seem to get very little deep sleep and spend most of their time alternating between light fitful sleep and REM sleep, even if they sleep for an adequate length of time. Many people also find they feel groggy if they try to sleep longer to catch up on lost sleep. Listen to what your body is telling you. If you find yourself yawning or falling asleep at nine o'clock, then go to bed. If you stay up for another half hour you may miss the key slot in your ultradian rhythm (*see* p.31). Getting up early should ensure you are ready for bed at a reasonable hour. Ayurvedic medicine suggests making your bedtime around 10pm, but whatever time you settle on, stick to it seven days a week.

Eating for peaceful sleep

A good diet is one of the most important factors in maintaining good health and sound sleep. Food affects our sleep in many ways. First of all it affects our health. Poor diet is a major factor in degenerative diseases such as cancer and heart disease. It is implicated in chronic conditions such as arthritis, allergies, diabetes, and digestive disorders and is also a factor in depression. In fact it is difficult to think of an illness that cannot be affected either beneficially or detrimentally by food. Any illness resulting in pain or discomfort will interfere with sleep and any pain or discomfort that can be alleviated by

Benefits of a low-fat diet

A low-fat, high-carbohydrate diet may help to relieve depression-related insomnia. In 1993 a study of 300 men and women found that depression and feelings of hostility dropped significantly and were replaced by enhanced psychological wellbeing in those who adopted a cholesterol-lowering diet.

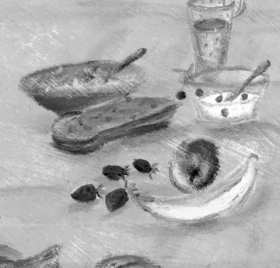

Breakfast

Breakfast is the most important meal of the day. When you get up early you are more likely to have the appetite for a fortifying and nutritious breakfast. Eat wholegrain bread and cereals, yoghurt, fruit, and fresh juice to maintain energy levels through the morning. Fruit, in particular, is an excellent breakfast food as it is full of vitamins and natural sugars that will increase your blood sugar levels.

Lunch

Opt for fruit, vegetables, and plenty of energy-giving complex carbohydrates. Choose wholegrain bread, brown rice, and pasta, in preference to refined products, to ensure sustained energy release over a longer period. Include only small amounts of proteins such as fish, chicken, eggs, meat, beans, and pulses. Proteins stimulate the production of dopamine, a chemical that is converted into adrenaline. Hence a little protein at lunchtime can power you through the afternoon.

Evening meal

Large late meals are not conducive to sleep. Eat a light meal at least two hours before bedtime. Choose complex carbohydrates such as pasta, brown rice, potatoes, and wholegrain bread, and combine them with eggs, dairy produce, and a little meat or fish, to produce the sedative amino acid tryptophan. Vegetarians can achieve the same results by combining complex carbohydrates with lentils and pulses. Fill up on vegetables and salads for light and refreshing evening eating that is easy to digest.

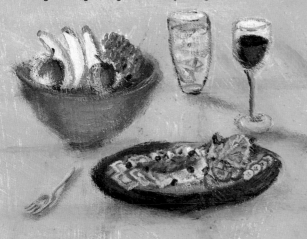

Alcohol

Although not recommended as a daily routine, the occasional tipple should do no harm to good sleepers. Taken in moderate amounts – a small measure of spirits, or one glass of wine with your evening meal, it can have a relaxing effect. Minimize its ill-effects by only drinking with or after a meal. Alcohol taken with food is absorbed more slowly into the bloodstream. Always remember that too much alcohol acts as a stimulant.

Daytime snacks

Fruit, sunflower seeds, and unsalted nuts help to maintain energy levels and mental alertness thanks to their boron and selenium content. Boron and selenium are trace minerals which studies have shown to leave you clear-headed and elated. Raisins also help to boost energy levels and tone the nervous system thanks to a substance called oenocyanine, which combines with dietary sugars to provide energy.

Late-night snacks

The contraction of an empty stomach can cause restless body movements and may even wake you up. Low blood sugar at night can disturb sleep by causing night sweats. A light snack before bedtime can prevent this from happening. Suitable late-night snacks include a soporific lettuce sandwich or a sandwich made from banana, avocado, or peanut butter, all of which are high in sleep-inducing tryptophan. A piece of toast and a glass of milk or a bowl of cereal are also good supper foods. Oatmeal porridge not only gives you energy in the morning, but helps to soothe an irritated nervous system at night. Likewise hot milky cereal drinks are beneficial. Oranges, especially mandarins, contain a sedative substance called bromine, making them ideal for soothing an over-excited nervous system.

dietary improvements will benefit sleep. Our energy and fitness levels depend on the food that fuels the body. Foods also have specific qualities. For example, some such as light proteins are energizing, others like lettuce and milky drinks have sedative qualities, and some such as refined sugars, caffeine, and an excess of salt are nutritionally empty and can be positively damaging to health.

What to eat when

The basic rules of a good health-giving diet also form the foundations of a healthy sleep diet. Fresh wholefoods – that is, foods that have had little or nothing added or taken away – should take the place of convenience foods overloaded with sugar, salt, and saturated fats. Choose plenty of vegetables, fruit, wholegrain cereals, breads, pasta, and rice, and moderate amounts of lean meat such as chicken and fish cakes, in preference to pastries, white bread, prepacked meals, processed and canned produce, sugary foods and drinks, fatty red meat, and prepared meat products. Cook-chill foods, microwave meals, and "fast" foods such as hamburgers, pizzas, and chips (French fries) are fine occasionally, but they should not be considered the basis of a healthy diet.

Vitamin B

Deficiency of B vitamins, which are found in a wide variety of wholegrain cereals, is linked to stress and insomnia. The risk of deficiency of this group of vitamins is increased if your diet is high in products made with white flour, which has had its B vitamins removed. Stress also uses up B vitamins. B vitamins are needed for a healthy nervous system. The B vitamins work in a delicate balance, so if you do take a supplement make sure it includes all of the B-complex vitamins.

Stimulants in food

Starch, sugar, and salt can keep you lying awake. Salt has been implicated as a cause of insomnia and salt-based flavourings, such as monosodium glutamate, appear to stimulate nerve endings, leading to hyperactivity and an inability to get to sleep. Over-consumption of sugar has also been blamed as a cause of hyperactivity in children.

Food additives in the form of chemical colourings, flavourings, and preservatives are in every processed food. Most food additives are safe, but some have been implicated in hyperactivity. Artificial sweeteners such as aspartame, and some food colourings (notably tartrazine) are among the worst. Children are particularly vulnerable because their immune systems are not fully developed.

Get active

People who do physical work outdoors – for example farmers, fishermen, construction workers, and forest rangers may find they get enough fresh air and exercise to leave them craving sleep at the end of the day. But if you have a sedentary job you are unlikely to get enough aerobic exercise unless you cycle to work or make regular trips to the gym. Sitting in an office can be mentally exhausting, but leaves you physically under-used. This imbalance between mind and body frequently manifests itself as disturbed or restless sleep. Lack of exercise also leads to excess weight and slack muscles, the forerunners to snoring and sleep apnoea. Regular exercise, on the other hand, tones muscles, boosts the immune system, and helps to fight depression.

Sleep is a natural response to physical tiredness. By building regular exercise into your daily routine, you are likely to increase your amount of deep sleep, during which the highest levels of growth hormone are released. Twenty to 30 minutes of vigorous exercise taken regularly benefits both mental and physical health.

Choose a form of exercise you enjoy and that you can do without strain or injury. Swimming and walking are both excellent aerobic activities, suitable for people of all ages and levels of fitness. Ayurvedic experts say you can avoid injury and exhaustion by exercising to half of your capacity. For example, if you know that jogging for 20 minutes will exhaust you jog for only ten. If your fitness level improves to the point where you could jog for 30 minutes, only do it for 15. The Chinese see exercise as a way of rebalancing the energies of body, mind, and spirit to maintain harmony and health. Systems such as *t'ai chi* and *qi qong* (pronounced "chee kung") look completely physically undemanding, but research shows that regular practice relaxes both muscular and nervous tension.

When to exercise

Morning, late afternoon, or early evening are all suitable times for all types of exercise. The time to avoid strenuous exercise is late at night. Leave at least two hours between any vigorous physical activity and bedtime. However, some forms of gentle exercise, such as yoga, can be built in to your pre-sleep routine (*see* Chapter Ten).

Chapter Nine

Your sleep environment

Your bedroom should be a peaceful haven with an atmosphere that seduces you into a deep relaxing sleep. It is somewhere to unwind, be intimate, and shut out the rest of the world. Everything about the room, the temperature, the type of mattress you use, the colour, and even where you place your bed is vitally important to enable you to sleep peacefully. There are many ways to get a better night's sleep, but the best place to start is by making your own bedroom a more restful place to be.

Where to place your bedroom

The first thing that you should attend to is the position of your bedroom in the home. Of course not all of us have the luxury of having a choice in this matter, but it may be worth considering these factors when choosing a new home. Common sense suggests that a room at the back of the house, away from the noise of traffic and the glare of street lamps, is the best place for those whose sleep is easily disrupted.

You should also give attention to the north-south orientation of the windows in your bedroom; children may be best suited to bedrooms in which the windows are facing east, so they enjoy the strength of the rising sun's energizing force, whereas older people may benefit more from a west-facing window through which the gentle rays of the setting sun have a calming influence. If a bedroom window is south facing, it wastes all the benefits of the sun's light and energy as most bedrooms are not occupied for most of the day.

"Sick" bedrooms

Those who work in modern office buildings commonly suffer from a variety of symptoms – known collectively as "sick building syndrome". These symptoms, such as nausea, depression, headaches, breathing problems, and fatigue, are thought to be the result of the effects of electrical equipment and synthetic fabrics and furnishings. To a lesser degree, your bedroom may also be "sick" enough to affect your health and the quality of your sleep.

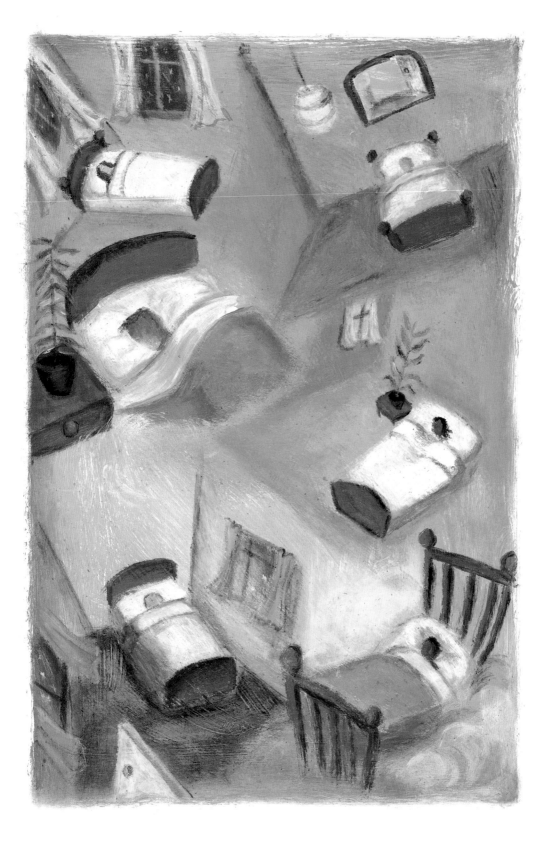

Feng shui in the bedroom

Feng shui (pronounced fung shoy) is the traditional Chinese art and science of home design. The ancient Chinese believed that the earth, the atmosphere, and every person or object on the earth affects and is affected by the flow of universal energy or *qi*. Feng shui practitioners aim to position buildings and the rooms and furniture within them in a way that enables us to live in harmony with the lines of energy that run through the earth. The theory of feng shui has much in common with the principles of geomancy, the study of how the earth's electromagnetic energy and its flow through ley lines affects our lives, and how their adverse effects can cause geopathic stress (see below). However, the earth's natural energy is also considered a powerful healing force. The key is to be able to avoid the stressed areas and tap into its healing benefits. The best way to apply the principles of feng shui is to have a professional consultant come to your home and assess your needs.

Sleep quality in polar regions

A study on men working in the polar regions found that they had little deep sleep as a result of the polar magnetic field. Not until a year after they returned home did their sleep habits return to normal.

Geopathic stress

Geopathic stress is the name given to the natural and artificial electromagnetic forces that surround us. This energy includes forces generated by the earth itself. The forces are most obvious in areas above an underground stream, near geological faults in the earth's crust, and near deeply excavated areas such as mines. Electromagnetic energy is also generated by electricity pylons, radios, televisions, and computers. Together these forces can have a damaging effect on our health.

Regular exposure to geopathic stress, like all forms of stress, can undermine the immune system and disrupt body functioning. In those people who are particularly sensitive it is believed to contribute to symptoms ranging from insomnia and sleepwalking to depression, high blood pressure, and even cancer. In terms of sleep disturbance, insomnia, teeth grinding, sleep-walking, and feeling cold or restless in bed, are all considered signs of geopathic stress. Since we spend around a third of our time asleep in bed, it is worth making sure that the bedroom is free from geopathic stress. Areas of geopathic stress can be very small and simply moving your bed to another part of the room may be all it takes to reduce their effect. Professional dowsers or kinesiologists can detect areas of geopathic stress using simple testing procedures.

Creating a sanctuary

Take a good look at your bedroom and ask yourself if it really is a place of rest, relaxation, and intimacy. Bedrooms are not for work or worry, they should be for sleep and sex only. The bedroom is one of the few places where you should be completely relaxed and alone, or intimate with a partner. If your bedroom is not only for sleeping in but also serves as an office and all-purpose dumping ground it is time to make changes.

Feng shui teaches that the single most important remedy for the home is to clear it of clutter. For greater peace of mind, sell, give away, or recycle unwanted possessions. Work-related items, computers, and electrical equipment should be removed from the bedroom. Televisions are not only visually stimulating, they also emit electromagnetic radiation, which is bad for health. The more electrical devices you can get rid of the better. Replace mains-operated radios with battery-operated models and use manual alarm clocks. If you live in a bedsit, studio flat, or large open-plan space, use a screen, curtain or book-case to divide your bed from your work area or make a symbolic division using mirrors, mobiles, or plants.

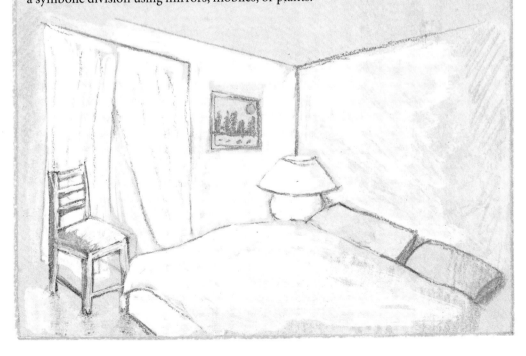

Your bedroom design

There are numerous ways in which you can improve the design of your sleep environment to encourage sounder sleep, but do not try to make too many changes at once and do not change anything that you are already happy with. Not all the suggestions on the following pages will appeal or be practicable for everyone, but giving your bedroom a rethink can often produce a noticeable change in your quality of sleep.

Plants

Houseplants help to remove air pollutants, and although they remove oxygen at night, their environmental benefits outweigh this disadvantage.

Doors

The relationship between the door and your bed is central to how your bedroom feels. Position your bed so that you can see the door, but you are not directly in front of its invading energy. If this is not possible, hang wind chimes between the bed and the door to create a symbolic division.

Ventilation

Cross-ventilation is the most effective way of cooling a hot or stuffy room. Open windows in more than one wall of your bedroom, or open a bedroom window, leave your bedroom door open, and open a window at the other side of the building to draw the ventilation through your room.

Flooring

Wooden or cork floors are less likely to harbour allergenic dust than carpets. For comfort, choose cotton rugs that can be washed regularly.

Mirrors

Mirrors in bedrooms can have an unsettling effect because they intensify the energy reflected in them You should not place a mirror opposite your bed as it reflects stimulating energy back towards your bed at night. If it is difficult to find a suitable spot for your mirror, it is best to conceal it inside a cupboard or wardrobe or cover it at night.

Windows

Have heavy curtains to keep out unwanted noise and light. Double-glazing can also be helpful if loud noise is a problem.

Bed

Feng shui recommends that you do not sleep with the head of your bed against or underneath a window, as the area behind your head should be solid if it is to give you a feeling of security and allow you to relax.

Lighting

During the time that you are asleep it is best to keep your bedroom as dark as possible. Feng shui experts would suggest moving your bed out of the path of direct sunlight, as sunlight is associated with daytime and activity and disturbs sleep. The type of lighting in your bedroom and where the lights are positioned can also affect how you feel when you are in that room. Soft lighting from different sources such as a bedside lamp and uplighters on the walls are more restful than the glare of a central bulb.

Storage

Keep clothes and other possessions stored out of sight in closed cupboards to minimize visual "noise".

Ionizers

Ionizers are electrical devices that emit negative ions to help clear the air of dust, smoke, and some allergens. Ions are positive and negatively electrically charged molecules. A healthy balance of positive and negative ions promotes feelings of calm and wellbeing. However, central heating, electrical appliances, synthetic fabrics, pollution and dust all deplete levels of negative ions, which can contribute to headaches, irritability, and general feelings of discomfort.

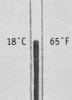

18°C   65°F

Temperature

For most people a temperature of around 18°C (65°F) is most conducive to restful sleep. In order to maintain a comfortable temperature in winter, it is usually necessary to heat the room throughout the night.

Finding the right bed

Since most of us spend a third of our life in bed it can be considered the most important piece of furniture in the home. While the recommended life span for a bed is ten years, the average person keeps theirs for more than 17 years, putting up with increasingly uncomfortable nights as it becomes less firm, more lumpy, and saggy in the middle. In the first scientific survey of its kind, French researchers reported that even poor sleepers got to sleep more quickly, woke up less during the night, and accumulated almost an extra hour of sleep in a new bed compared to one that was ten years old.

We each have different needs when it comes to choosing a bed. A thinner person may want a slightly softer bed for more cushioning, while someone with back problems needs a firm or orthopaedic mattress. Some couples prefer to have adjoining twin beds that can be individually adjusted, rather than the conventional double.

Choosing a mattress

A good mattress is essential for good quality sleep. As a general rule, the more expensive, the better the quality, but decide which gives most comfort and support. It is not true that firm mattresses are better. A bed that is too hard may cause just as many problems as a soft or lumpy bed. When trying one out, lie down and slide the flat of your hand under the small of your back. If you have to wedge it between the mattress and your back, it's too soft; if there's a hollow, it's too hard.

You also need to decide on which type of interior you prefer. Ask about the fillings and check that the inner layers are able to act as a good drain for the pint or more of body moisture we lose during sleep each night. Most mattresses have metal springs. It is generally believed the more springs the better the bed, but springs are also believed to exacerbate the effects of electromagnetic radiation. Because they are metal, springs act as magnets that distort the earth's natural magnetic fields and can lead to

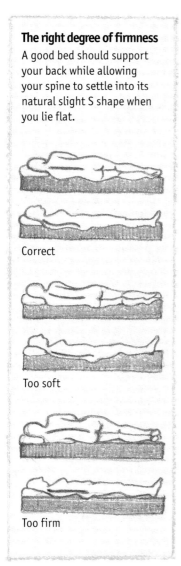

The right degree of firmness
A good bed should support your back while allowing your spine to settle into its natural slight S shape when you lie flat.

Correct

Too soft

Too firm

electrostress. If you want to avoid sprung mattresses there is the option of polyurethane foam mattresses, which are flexible and hard-wearing. Mattresses made from latex, a substance derived from the sap of rubber trees, can be expensive, but are comfortable and durable and do not need to be turned. Other new mattresses need to be turned end to end and side to side every month for the first six months and then at least once a year after that.

The advantages of futons

Futons are traditional Japanese mattresses made from natural fabrics. Natural calico covers are filled with layers of cotton and wool wadding and the mattress fits onto a slatted wooden base. Futons have several benefits, principally that the slatted base provides good ventilation and reduces the build up of dust and other particles, so they are good for asthmatics and people with allergies. The all-natural fibres from which the mattress is made also allows air to circulate so that the skin breathes during sleep and the absence of metal springs reduces the risk of electromagnetic stress. Futons can be as comfortable and supportive as any good bed. They have a shorter life span than a conventional bed, about four or five years, but they cost a fraction of the price of a quality sprung mattress.

Size of bed
Beds should be at least 15cm (6in) longer than the occupants, with doubles being at least 135cm (4ft 6in) wide and singles at least 90cm (3ft) wide. This allows space to move and extra room to stretch out as the spine, which contracts during the day, lengthens by about 2cm (1in) during the night.

Sleeping position
The direction in which your head lies may influence your sleep. Charles Dickens always slept with his head pointing north – even if it meant moving the furniture. However, others, such as those following yogic traditions, believe that pointing north has a bad effect and that sleeping with the head towards the east is best.

The Chinese believe that the best way to sleep is on your right side with your legs slightly bent and your right arm bent and resting in front of the pillow. The left arm should rest on the left thigh. In this position blood can circulate freely and the *hun* (ethereal soul – *see* p.18) remains firmly footed in the liver.

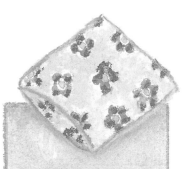

Pillows for sound sleep

Your head accounts for one fifth of your body weight, so it needs to be well supported when lying down. A good pillow keeps the head in the same relation to your shoulders and spine as when you are standing up. The type of pillow you choose may depend on how you sleep. If you prefer lying on your back when you drop off, try a medium-firm pillow, which will "give" as you sleep. If you sleep on your side, you need to support your head and neck with a firm pillow. If you sleep on your stomach a soft pillow will cause less strain on your neck.

Most pillows are now made with synthetic fibres or foams. These are good for those with allergies and can easily be washed in a washing machine. Down or feather pillows are more luxurious, but are suitable only for people who are not allergic to feathers.

Herb pillows

Some people like to use a small hop or herb filled pillow along with their usual pillow to induce restful sleep. Herbs have well-documented thera-peutic properties, but their effects can be nullified if the smell irritates you, so sniff well before you buy.

Bedclothes

Maintaining a comfortable temperature is vital for sound sleep and bedclothes therefore have an important role in ensuring sleep quality. Most people use duvets these days as they provide warmth without the weight of blankets, and they make bedmaking faster. However, you cannot add to them or take away to compensate for changes in room temperature in the same way as you can with blankets, so for some people blankets are still preferable. Many duvet manufac-turers now produce all-season duvets. These usually comprise a pair of duvets of different weights, which snap together to provide extra warmth in winter and can be used individually as a cooler covering in summer. Natural fabrics and fillings are usually better than synthetics as they let your skin breathe. However, synthetic fillings are preferable for people who are allergic to feathers. Duvets are not suitable for babies: soft cotton sheets and cotton cellular blankets are the best bedding for cots (cribs).

Keeping warm in bed

One of the easiest ways of staying warm in bed is to wear more clothes. Natural fabrics such as cotton and wool are effective insulators that allow the skin to breathe. It is also easier to stay warm if the bed is warm when you get into it. Place a hot water bottle in the bed about 30 minutes before you go to bed, but remove it before you get into bed. Avoid using electric blankets, because they emit electromagnetic radiation (p.105).

Colour choices in the bedroom

Doctors and psychologists, as well as colour therapists, agree that colour can greatly affect mood and behaviour. Intuitively, we describe our feelings in terms of colour. The expressions "seeing red", "feeling blue", or "going green with envy" are apt indications of how colour affects the emotions. An American study of the moods of prisoners found that they became much calmer and more controllable when their cell walls were painted a delicate shade of pink. If colour can have such a dramatically soothing effect on hardened criminals it's not surprising that the colour of your bedroom can influence the quality of your sleep.

Colour affects each of us individually, but there are general guidelines about colour qualities and how the different shades and tones of a particular colour can change a room. According to feng shui soft tones are best for the bedroom. Warm pinks, soft peaches, calm creams, relaxing pale greens, and even pale mauves and lilacs are restful bedroom choices.

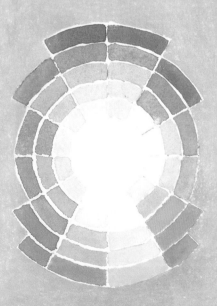

Pinks Warm pinks and peach tones are among the most restful colours for the bedroom.

Yellows and earth tones Strong yellows, oranges, and browns are too active to be suitable for bedrooms, although pale yellows and beiges are restful.

Greens Pale greens can be soothing in the bedroom, but darker tones may be oppressive.

Blues Feng shui practitioners tend to avoid the use of blue in decoration, yet some colour therapists believe blue, particularly pale, lilac shades can be restful and calming in bedrooms.

Reds Red, which is vibrant and stimulating (it has been found to speed up the circulation and raise blood pressure), is a colour to avoid if you want to enjoy peaceful sleep.

Avoiding allergens in the bedroom

Allergies can make it difficult to get to sleep because of feelings of discomfort or anxieties about not being able to breathe well. Allergic symptoms occur when your body reacts abnormally to something. Touching or even just breathing in small amounts of these substances, or allergens, causes the body to react, producing symptoms such as sneezing, an itchy, congested, or runny nose, streaming eyes, headaches, and even mild depression. Breathing difficulty is a common symptom, which can also cause snoring and you may wake up during the night with the sensation that you cannot breathe. Doctors prescibe antihistamine drugs to control allergies, but prevention is the healthier alternative to suppressing the symptoms.

Many of the common triggers of allergic reactions are found in the bedroom so it makes sense to ensure that your sleep environment is as allergen free as possible.

House-dust mite

Invisible to the naked eye, this tiny insect can cause allergies and asthma. The mites thrive in warm, moist conditions, so beds are their ideal homes, although they also inhabit carpets, soft toys, curtains, and upholstery. It is not the mite, but its droppings, that are highly allergenic, and some experts believe they are responsible for nearly half of all cases of asthma.

Even the cleanest of houses contains dust mites, but you can keep them to a minimum by vacuuming the whole room regularly – carpet, mattress, curtains and drapes, furnishings. Vacuums that have a high level of filtration recirculate less dust. Ventilation is also essential, and a dry, well-ventilated room with the minimum of central heating deters the mites.

Other measures include reducing the amount of soft furnishings in the room. If you are badly affected, consider removing your bedroom carpet and replacing it with a wooden floor, or cork or other non-synthetic tiles. Wash bedding regularly and at a high temperature, and replace old pillows and mattresses with new ones. Specialist anti-allergy bed covers can also help to keep the mites at bay.

The effects of household chemicals

Choose cleaning products and other household items carefully. Products such as cleaning agents, polish, bleach, disinfectant, and air-fresheners may all cause allergies. Symptoms can range from headache to fatigue, nausea, rhinitis, wheezing, coughing, eczema, and urticaria (hives). Where you can, use alternatives. Buy pure beeswax polish for furniture and wooden floors instead of chemical spray polishes, use biodegradable cleaners for paintwork and surfaces, or use vinegar or a baking soda solution to clean and disinfect surfaces. If you decide to use chemical sprays and cleaning products in your bedroom, open the windows while you clean so that their toxic vapours can escape.

Beds and furniture made from chipboard, hardboard, and fibreboard can emit formaldehyde as can carpets, upholstery, and bedding. Formaldehyde, which is used as an industrial binder and preservative, is present in numerous household products from fabrics to cosmetics and is a known irritant and suspected carcinogen. You can buy low-emission formaldehyde boards or simply buy or make furniture from solid, natural wood instead.

Where possible beds and furniture should be made from untreated solid timber or cane and bedding and furnishings from untreated cotton, linen, and wool. Wash all bedding before you use it, because even natural fabrics may have been chemically cleaned, bleached, and coloured unless otherwise stated. Houseplants, especially the common spider plant, are surprisingly effective at removing formaldehyde from the atmosphere.

Other pollutants

Animal dander (skin flakes) is a common allergen. The bedroom is no place for animals, and people who let their pet share their room should seriously reconsider the health implications of this habit. Moulds grow in warm, damp areas and release allergy-provoking spores. Keep the room clean, dry, and well ventilated. The risks of cigarette smoke are well known. Keep smoke out of the house and definitely out the bedroom.

Chapter Ten

Your pre-sleep routine

Sleep is the end-product of a gradual winding down process. Setting aside a sleep preparation time gets us in the mood for bed and helps us to make the gradual transition from a day filled with activity, stress, and stimulation, to a calm and relaxed evening.

Everyone has their own pre-sleep routine. If you have one that works for you then stick with it. But people with sleep problems often have no recognizable routine or have one that simply does not work. If sleep is a problem for you, take a look at your habits in the hours before bedtime. Make a list of all the things you do in the evening when you come home from work. Jot down what time you start and finish each activity and when you have read this chapter you can decide if your own evening routine is helping or hindering your sleep.

The recommendations in this chapter are suggestions rather than a complete prescription for preparing yourself for sleep. You do not have to follow every item of advice: you may need to make only one or two changes to notice a difference in the quality of your sleep.

Make the break

Making a break between daytime activities and the inactivity associated with night helps to encourage sleep. If you are worried about a work project, money, or afraid of forgetting an important appointment, it is often difficult to stop yourself worrying during the evening and into the night. One way to make it easier is to write down everything that is preying on your mind. Do this when

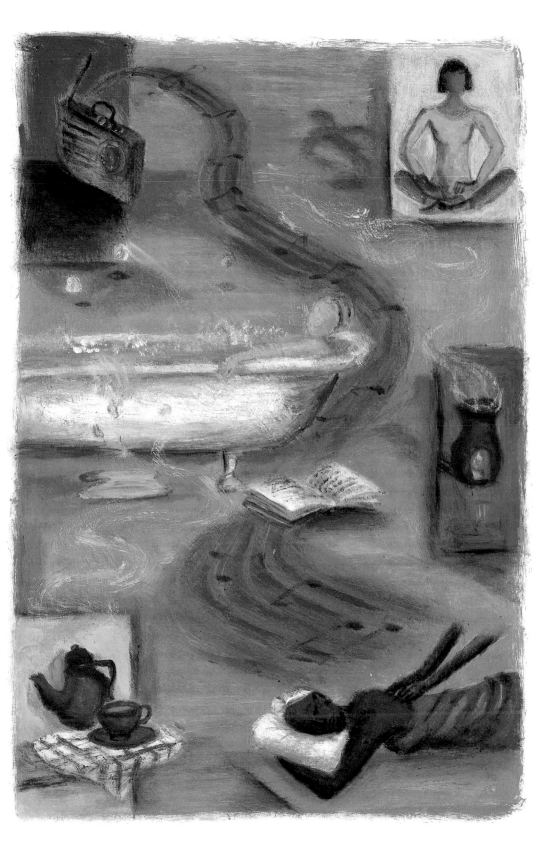

you come home from work or after you have finished the main activities of the day. The list should be a review of the day's events and a plan for the following day. When problems are written down they somehow seem smaller and more manageable. If there is anything you can resolve straight away, do it and get it out of the way. If there is nothing you can do until the next day, accept this and forget about it.

Relax and unwind

Relaxation is vital to restful sleep and there are many ways to unwind. Relaxation is not about slumping in front of the television after eating a huge meal. In fact, most forms of beneficial relaxation involve working with your mind and body to let go of tension. This may sound like a contradiction, but gentle systems of exercise such as yoga and *t'ai chi* have been shown to relieve muscular tension and mental stress. Yoga can have an energizing effect, but the

Relaxation tapes

Pre-recorded relaxation tapes or CDs can be helpful. Although each may offer slightly differing methods of relaxation, such as visualization, self-hypnosis, or muscle relaxation, the end result should be the same – a soothed mind and body, ready for sleep.

Progressive relaxation technique

This simple technique can help reduce tension and knotted muscles and release the body from pain.

♦ Lie or sit with your eyes closed in a dark room. Starting at your toes, tense your muscles, hold for the count of three, then relax them.

♦ Tense and release all the major muscle groups in the body, working from your toe and finger tips up to your neck and facial muscles.

♦ Breathe deeply as you do it, take a slow breath in through the nose, hold for the count of five, then exhale slowly through the mouth while repeating the word "calm" in your mind.

Passive muscular relaxation

This is a variation that can be practised by people with physical disabilities, who may have problems tensing muscles. Instead of tensing a muscle group you simply focus your attention on it, acknowledge the tension already there and then release it. You can help the relaxation process by imagining a slow, warm wave of relaxation washing through your muscles, lengthening and expanding them and freeing any knots or tensions.

gentle stretches described in Part Four make up a relaxing sequence, specially designed to encourage sleep.

T'ai chi, meaning wholeness, is an ancient Chinese system of exercise. The exercises consist of a series of slow, graceful, dance-like movements, commonly referred to as "mediation in motion". The fluid movements of *t'ai chi* help to alleviate anxiety, stress, and the emotional anguish that can lead to insomnia. It is not possible to learn *t'ai chi* effectively without the guidance of an experienced teacher, but if there are classes available in your area, it would be worthwhile to give them a try.

If these forms of exercise do not appeal, a gentle walk – for example, to exercise the dog – could provide an effective alternative. A variety of other self-help techniques can also help to relax mind and body. These include progressive relaxation, meditation, biofeedback, and the visualization and breathing exercises described on p.123.

Biofeedback

This relaxation technique is sometimes taught in sleep clinics. Medical monitoring equipment is used to measure heart rate, blood pressure, muscle tension, skin temperature, sweat, and blood flow through the hands and feet. The monitors enable you to see how your body systems react to stress or the lack of it. Providing this sort of feedback can help you to recognize when you are stressed and enable you to learn to reduce tension in yourself.

Meditation

Meditation is a form of deep relaxation that allows your whole body to rest while your mind stays in a state of "relaxed alertness". You need no special gifts or talents to meditate. You simply need to be prepared to practise for about 15 minutes every day. There are many different ways to meditate. A simple meditation exercise is described here.

♦ You need a warm and quiet environment and a "mantra" – an object or word on which to focus. This can be your breath, which you count each time you exhale, or a word that has no psychological associations.

♦ Sit in a comfortable position on a cushion on the floor or on a straight-backed chair with your hands resting in your lap or on your knees.

♦ Close your eyes, relax, and breathe deeply and regularly through your nose.

♦ Focus on your breath, counting each breath as you exhale. It is common to count to ten and repeat, but beginners may find it easier to count to four.

♦ Don't attempt to modify your breathing, or think about anything other than counting each breath as you exhale.

♦ When your mind wanders (and it will), calmly return your attention to your breath. Don't try to stop other thoughts, just acknowledge them and let them go. At the end of the meditation, stretch and get up slowly.

The hour before sleep

You have put the day's worries behind you, had a nourishing but not heavy meal, and done some form of relaxing exercise. In the hour or so before actually going to bed concentrate on pleasurable, pampering activities that are designed to soothe your mind and body into a state of readiness for sleep.

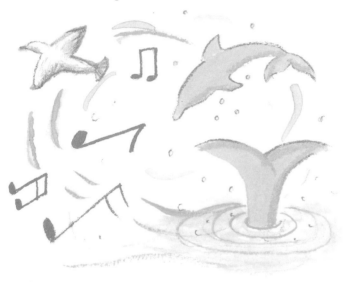

Natural sleep remedies

If you feel that you need to take a natural sleep remedy, do so about half an hour before bedtime. Herbal or homeopathic remedies that you can buy from health food stores, herbalists, or pharmacies can help with sleep problems. Treat all sleep remedies with caution, read the dosage instructions, and take them only for as long as you need. Natural sleep remedies are discussed more fully in Part Four.

The relaxing power of music

Music can alter our moods, relax our senses, and soothe muscles as tension ebbs out with the flow of sound. Which kind of music you choose is up to you, but gentle melodious pieces are more caressing than rock music. Alternatively, you could listen to natural sounds, such as dolphin and whale music, lapping waves, or birdsong.

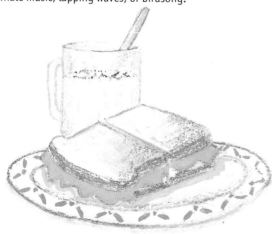

Snacks and nightcaps

Some people find it comforting to eat a little before bedtime. The golden rule with food is to keep it light and aim for foods that have sleep-inducing qualities (*see* Chapter Eight). Drinks should also be chosen for their sedative benefits. The success of the traditional warm, milky bedtime drink may in part be due to its tryptophan content. This amino acid is a constituent of serotonin, from which the sleep hormone melatonin is derived.

A bath before bedtime

A bath is much more relaxing than a shower, and the warm water raises body temperature so that you feel more inclined to sleep. Keep the water temperature slightly warmer than your own body temperature, but do not make it too hot as this can leave you feeling weak and sweaty, and dilates the blood vessels, putting a strain on your heart. Don't stay in a hot bath more than about 15 minutes or you risk becoming overheated. Make your bathtime special. Add a favourite bubble bath or a few drops of aromatherapy oil. Choose those with soothing and relaxing properties from the selection given in Part Four. Close the door to keep the vapours in and everybody else out.

Late-night reading and watching television

Reading and watching television are not ideal late-evening activities for those with sleep problems, but for many people they form part of the pre-sleep ritual. The activity itself is not conducive or detrimental to sleep, it depends on what you read or watch that determines the night ahead. Stick to these basic rules when choosing your late-night reading or viewing:

Reading

♦ Never read anything related to work, especially in bed.
♦ Don't read exciting books that you won't be able to put down.
♦ Don't shut the book on a cliff-hanger.
♦ Don't fall asleep trying to finish a chapter or reach the end.
♦ Avoid horror stories or thrillers that can keep you awake or give you nightmares.

Television

♦ Keep the television out of the bedroom.
♦ Avoid stimulating or frightening programmes that may keep you awake or give you nightmares.
♦ Don't start to watch a programme that finishes way past your usual bedtime.
♦ Don't fall asleep in front of the television.

Going to bed

Go to bed when you are sleepy, taking advantage of the natural ultradian cycles of drowsiness (*see* Chapter Two), and not before. If you go to bed as soon as you feel tired you should fall asleep quite easily, but if you delay, the sleepiness will pass and you'll feel wide awake again. Once in bed, you could try self-hypnosis or another sleep-inducing technique. Self-hypnosis is described in more detail on p.140.

Sex is a great aid to sleep if you have a willing partner. Humans thrive on touch and sex can provide a closeness and warmth that can make other problems fade into the background until morning. Evidence also suggests that sex itself has a beneficial effect on our ability to sleep – which is why we tend to roll over and fall asleep afterward. A bedtime massage can also help, not only by putting you in the mood for sex, but also by calming the nervous system. You could try a sleep-inducing shiatsu massage on the pressure points associated with sleep (*see* facing page).

If you cannot sleep

If when you go to bed you find yourself unable to sleep, get up and do something boring until you feel sleepy again. Lying awake in bed only increases your anxiety about not sleeping, which in turn contributes to sleeplessness. When you feel sleepy again go back to bed and try again. Alternatively, you could try some sleep-promoting exercises such as visualization or the Ayurvedic technique described on p.123.

Sleep-restriction therapy

This therapy has helped many people to relearn that a bed is for sleeping in and not for lying awake thinking about it. The idea is to keep the total amount of time you spend in bed nearly equal to the amount of time you spend asleep. So, do not go to bed until you feel sleepy. If you go to bed and do not fall asleep within 20 minutes get up and do something else until you feel sleepy again.

Don't go to bed angry

Anger is a destructive emotion that, among its many other damaging effects, can prevent you from getting to sleep. Do not start an argument just before bedtime as you will be too agitated to sleep. If you have a problem, worry, or complaint sort it out before bedtime or write it down and decide to deal with it the next day. Do not take your problems to bed with you, they do not make good bedfellows.

Shiatsu massage for sleep

This Japanese system of massage identifies particular points for sleep-inducing massage. Gentle but firm pressure with the thumb in each of the areas (known as *tsubos*) shown can be helpful for some people.

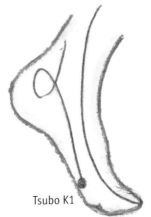

Tsubo GV 20

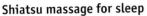

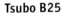

Tsubo B25

Tsubo GV 20

Use both thumbs to press firmly downward for 10 to15 seconds at the centre of the head at the point in line with the upper edge of the ears.

Tai yo

Press with one thumb for seven to ten seconds on points about one finger's width to the side of each eyebrow, between the end of the eyebrow and the outer edge of the eye.

Tsubo B25

Press three times for five to seven seconds on the points about 4cm (1½ in) to either side between the fouth and fifth lumbar vertebrae.

Tsubo K1

Tsubo K1

Use both thumbs to press hard and inward for 10 to 15 seconds on a point on the sole of the foot about a third of the distance from the tip of the middle toe to the heel, between the second and third toe joints.

Then go back to bed and start again. People who believe that they lie awake for hours before getting to sleep can benefit from restricting their time in bed to only a few hours for the first few nights. This ensures that you are so tired you quickly fall asleep once in bed. It also helps to create a new perception of yourself as someone who goes to bed and sleeps. As your sleep improves you can gradually increase your time in bed, so you eventually work your way round to going to bed and having a full night's sleep. Remember, a full night's sleep is not necessarily eight hours. If you find you only sleep for six hours, stay in bed only for that amount of time.

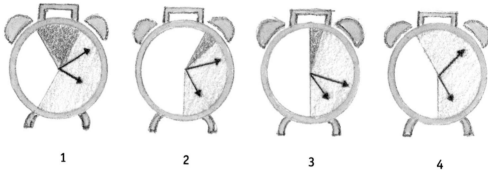

1   2   3   4

 In bed but awake

 Asleep

How to use sleep restriction therapy

1 Before therapy A person suffering from insomnia typically spends a long time in bed before they succeed in falling asleep.

2 First night of sleep restriction Do not go to bed until you feel sleepy. This may be several hours later than your usual bedtime. If when you go to bed, you cannot sleep within 20 minutes, get up and wait until you are even more sleepy before trying again. Set your alarm to wake you early in the morning, say at 6.30am, even if this means you get only a few hours sleep.

3 Second night Repeat the procedure for the first night, but go to bed somewhat earlier than you did the previous night. Get up at the same time the following morning.

4 Third and successive nights Maintain the principle of not going to bed until you are sleepy and getting up at a consistent, early time every morning. Gradually you should be going to bed at a regular time and sleeping soon after.

Get help if you need it

There are few sleep problems that cannot be overcome with self-help, careful planning, and commonsense. If you have tried all the recommendations in this book and you still cannot get the sleep you need, it is time to call in the professionals. Contact your doctor and ask to be referred to a sleep clinic, for counselling, or for an appropriate complementary therapy. Most general practitioners realize that sleep is essential if we are to remain healthy, well balanced, and productive.

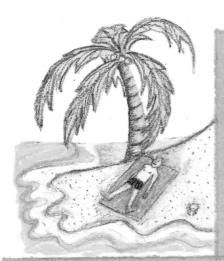

Visualization

If your mind is still racing as you lie in bed, try visualizing yourself basking in the most relaxing scenario imaginable. Choose a scene that is not only beautiful, but also devoid of stress. For example, if you love the sun and sea imagine yourself lying on a warm, peaceful exotic beach. Use all your senses to feel the sun on your face, smell the sea and sun lotion, taste the salt on your lips, and hear the waves gently lapping on the shore. Breathe slowly and deeply in time to the lapping waves, and allow yourself to drift off to sleep as if you were floating on top of warm waves.

Ayurvedic breathing exercise for insomnia

Try this exercise as an alternative to visualization. Lie down in bed with the light off and allow yourself to fall asleep while doing it.

♦ Focus on deep regular breathing for a few seconds.

♦ Give thanks for all the joys, experiences, even the trials of your day.

♦ Keeping an awareness of your breath, get into your most comfortable sleeping position.

♦ If you feel restless, just acknowledge that this excess *vata* energy will pass.

♦ Continue to breathe slowly and deeply. Try to imagine what your body feels like when it is in a deep relaxing sleep and allow yourself to drift into that sleepy state.

♦ If you wake in the night, do not get agitated, simply repeat the exercise.

Your sleep diary

Keeping a sleep diary should help to put your new healthy sleep regime into practice. It takes time to instigate lifestyle changes and reset body rhythms, and you may not see results for several weeks. Use a diary to monitor your progress over a five-week period. Be completely honest and stick to your routine. At the end of the fifth week review the situation to see how well you have progressed.

Date..

Bedtime.

.........am/pm

Wake-up time

.........am/pm

Did you drink alcohol or caffeine, or smoke tobacco within 4 hours of bedtime?

yes/no
Specify type and quantity
....

Did you take sleeping pills?

yes/no
Specify type and quantity
....

Did you use a natural remedy?

yes/no
Specify type and quantity
....

Did you take other medication within 4 hours of bedtime?

yes/no
Specify type and quantity
....

Did you exercise during the day?

yes/no
When and for how long
....

Did you use any relaxation technique or massage?

yes/no
What did you use and when
....

Did you nap during the day?

yes/no
Number ....
For how long ....

Keep a record of each day's activities and other information that may be relevant to the amount and quality of sleep you achieve each night. This page can be photocopied for use as your daily sleep record.

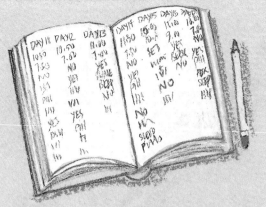

How quickly did you fall asleep at night?

less than 15 min
15-30 min
30-45 min
45-60 min
more than 60 min

How frequently did you wake during the night?

not at all
once
2-3 times
4-5 times
6 or more times ......

How much sleep did you get in total during the night?

less than 4 hrs
4-5 hrs
5-6 hrs
6-7 hrs
more than 7hrs

How good was your sleep?

great / good / average / poor / terrible

How did you feel in the morning?

great / good / average / poor / terrible

How much of the basic advice in Part Three of this book did you follow?

most / some / a little / none

Do you think your sleep has improved?

yes/no

Which aspect of your sleep has improved most?

Describe ....

Which aspect has improved least?

Describe ....

Do you think you need professional help?

yes/no

Chapter Eleven

A place for pills?

When you consider how common sleep disorders are among adults it is not surprising that sleeping pills are big business. But the irony is that as more sleeping pills have become available increasing numbers of people are claiming to suffer from insomnia. There may be many reasons for this: we may be more inclined to seek medical help for insomnia than our parents and grandparents did, or more people may be developing insomnia as a direct result of high stress levels. There is no clear explanation for the increase or for the fact that more women than men take sleeping pills.

The effects of sleeping pills

Most people fall asleep within an hour of taking a sleeping drug. However, the sleep they get is not like normal sleep. Most sleeping drugs induce sleep by depressing brain function as a whole. This interference with normal brain activity means that the quality of sleep produced is different from normal sleep. Most of us spend about a quarter of our total sleep time in REM sleep. When you first take sleeping pills REM can drop to as little as a tenth of total sleep time. However, if you continue to take the pills for a few weeks, the proportion of REM will gradually return to normal. The proportion of deep sleep is also seriously affected by sleeping drugs. It is not unusual for someone in a drug-induced sleep to spend as little as five per cent of total sleep time in deep sleep.

Sudden withdrawal from pills also has its problems. Most people who suddenly stop sleeping pills experience

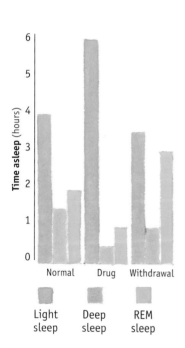

Drug-induced sleep

Drug-induced sleep differs from normal sleep. It contains a reduced proportion of both REM sleep and deep sleep. Sleep following the withdrawal of sleeping drugs contains a high proportion of REM sleep, leading to vivid dreams.

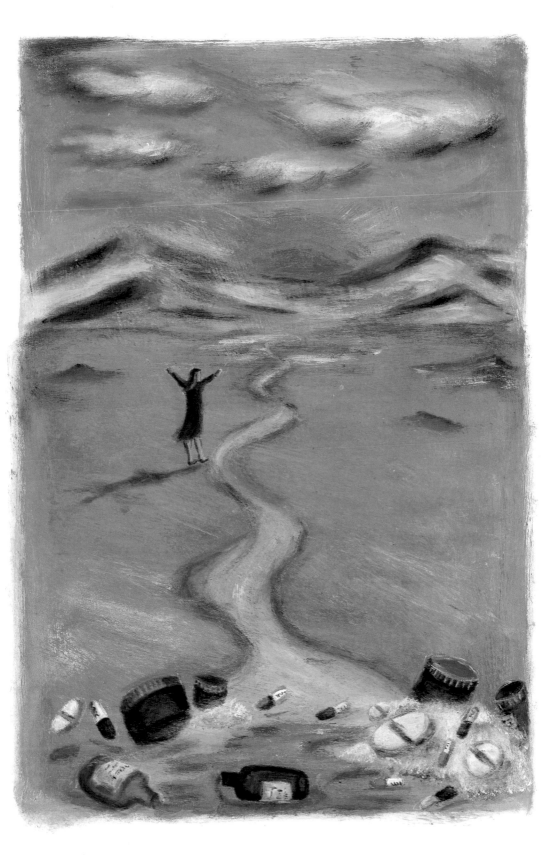

a rebound of REM sleep. Increased anxiety is also a common feature of sudden withdrawal, making it difficult to get to sleep and sleep through the night. These unpleasant withdrawal symptoms discourage many people from giving up sleeping pills long after they have ceased to have a useful effect.

Uses and limitations

Pills can be effective as a "quick fix", if no other immediate remedy is available on the odd night when lack of sleep can affect your performance the next day. They are beneficial for people who are over-anxious about a specific event and can also provide much needed relief from the exhaustion of an emotional trauma such as bereavement. Although sleeping pills can provide some respite from the pain of loss, they cannot hasten the grieving process, which is necessarily often long and difficult and may require specialist counselling.

While they can be effective as a temporary measure, drugs provide no solution to long-term sleeping problems. Insomnia caused by emotional stresses, such as marital problems, divorce, or financial crisis, are not resolved by taking a pill because sleeping drugs do not cure the problem, they simply help you to forget.

The pharmacological effect of sleeping pills wears off after two weeks because the body learns to tolerate them. But sleeping pills can also be addictive which is why many people continue to take them long after they have ceased to be beneficial. Over time regular users of sleeping pills may find that they remain stressed and anxious, but with the additional problem of a drug habit. The problem is exacerbated when people, finding that their usual dose no longer has any effect, take more in order to get to sleep.

Why the need for pills?

Bed can be a lonely place when it seems that all the world is asleep except you. The feelings of isolation and helplessness combined with anger at being awake when all you

Break the habit

If you want to break the cycle of taking sleeping pills start by believing that you can do it. For some it may be easy, with no apparent withdrawal symptoms. For others, symptoms may last a long time and be unpleasant, depending on the dosage and how long you've been taking them. But, rest assured, the symptoms will get better.

Forward planning

Make sure your partner, friends, or family know what you are about to undertake and are there for you. Enlist the help not only of your family doctor, but of other people you feel can help you, such as a counsellor or alternative therapist. Your doctor will be able to put you on a slow withdrawal programme and monitor your progress.

Choose the time

If you've got a particularly stressful event in the near future – you're moving house, getting married, divorced, or changing job – wait until it's quieter. On the other hand, don't keep putting it off until the next event arises. You can go through withdrawal and still cope with the normal stresses of life.

Ground rules

If you have been taking sleeping pills for less than two weeks you can stop as soon as you feel you no longer need them. But if you have taken them for longer, a programme of gradual withdrawal worked out with your doctor is necessary. Accept that it may take time, but that this gives your body a chance to get back to normal in a less shocking way. Remember it is normal to have ups and downs and try not to be disheartened by new symptoms. You should also be prepared to unearth and confront old emotional problems that may have led you to taking the pills in the first place.

The programme

You can reduce your nightly dose in stages every two to four weeks, depending on your progress. It may take several months to be completely free of the addiction. Use this time to look at other aspects of your health, to give yourself the best chance of total recovery.

♦ Cut down on caffeine and nicotine, but do not try to achieve too much at once. If you need all your energies to come off the pills, give up smoking some other time.

♦ Try to follow the advice in the previous chapters. Keep to regular hours of rising and going to bed, take some exercise, perhaps take up a new sport, or take up a new hobby.

♦ Pay special attention to your diet as you need all the nourishment you can get to keep strong and healthy. Make a point of cooking yourself a special meal at least once a week and try to enjoy great-tasting nutritious food whenever you can.

♦ Pamper yourself. Go for an aromatherapy massage; it not only feels relaxing and indulgent, but the therapist can use oils to relieve the symptoms of withdrawal.

want to do is sleep is enough in itself to keep many an insomniac tossing and turning.

There are many reasons why we accept taking sleeping pills. It can be easier to pop a pill than take a long hard look at the problems that are at the root of your insomnia. Several nights of transient insomnia can leave you desperate for a fast road to oblivion rather than face another sleepless night. Some people claim they are just too busy to spend the time it takes to revise their lifestyles, get in shape, and calm the stresses behind their sleeplessness. Others start taking pills in the belief that it will only be for a couple of days or weeks. Often this is the case and pills are a welcome – if short-lived – way of getting through the week. However, dependence grows very quickly and what started out as a stop-gap can quickly grow into a very unhealthy habit.

Natural alternatives

There are many useful, non-addictive sleep remedies that you can use as a temporary measure, if you prefer not to take pills. Part Four describes a full range of complementary therapies for sleeping problems. The following are natural compounds that have been found to be particularly beneficial alternatives to sleeping drugs.

♦ **Tryptophan** This amino acid, important for the repair of protein tissues and for creating new protein, is converted in the brain into serotonin, a natural sleep-inducing chemical. Taking a 1,000-1,500mg supplement before bed has been found to be helpful for some people. In Britain tryptophan tablets are only available on prescription, but the amino acid can also be found naturally in milk and carbohydrate and there is no risk associated with eating tryptophan-rich foods.

♦ **Melatonin** This is the sleep hormone. It is now being manufactured as a food supplement. Some studies have shown it to be beneficial for improving sleep and banishing jet lag. However, because its effects are not yet fully understood, pregnant or breast-feeding women, people under the age of 35, those with cancer of the blood or immune system, and those with kidney disease are advised not to take it. Synthetic melatonin may be safer than melatonin from animal sources. It should be taken at bedtime as it reaches peak concentration in the blood within an hour of consumption.

♦ **Kava Kava root** This herb is available as a food supplement. It has been found to depress the central nervous system and relax skeletal muscles, making it an effective mental and physical relaxant and an effective aid for the treatment of mild insomnia. The recommended dosage of standardized preparations is 100-200mg one hour before bedtime.

Group	Generic name(s) (common brands)	Effects	Risks
Benzodiazepines The most commonly used sleeping drugs	**chlordiazepoxide** *(Librium)* **diazepam** *(Valium)* **nitrazepam** *(Mogadon)* **temazepam** *(Normison, Restoril)*	Benzodiazepines work by depressing brain function. They interfere with chemical activity in the brain and nervous system by breaking down communication between the nerve cells. Reducing brain activity makes it easier to fall asleep.	Many people find they wake up feeling "hungover" and not as well rested as they would be with natural sleep. Effects are increased by drinking alcohol. There is a high risk of dependence with long-term use.
Benzodiazepine-like drugs The newest group of sleeping drugs	**zopiclone** *(Zimovane)* **zolpidem** *(Ambien, Stilnoct)*	These act at the same sites on nerve cells as benzodiazepines, but do not appear to affect the normal sleep pattern. The drugs take effect within 20-30 minutes and the effects last for six to eight hours. So far, tests show few "hangover" effects the following day.	It is still not certain what level of tolerance there is to them or what withdrawal symptoms may develop. Dizziness and poor co-ordination may be temporary problems. There have been occasional reports of hallucinations, forgetfulness, and behavioural disturbances such as aggression, but mostly in people who already had a history of benzodiazepine or other drug abuse.
Antihistamines These drugs are more commonly used in the prevention and treatment of allergies	**promethazine** *(Phenergan)* **trimeprazine** *(Vallergan)*	Sometimes used for sleep problems, mainly in children. They are also beneficial if allergic symptoms are keeping you awake, but can take a long time to act so should be taken early in the evening. Their sleep-inducing effect is produced by their depressant effect on the brain.	May cause dizziness and affect co-ordination, leading to clumsiness. Side effects can include nausea, dry mouth, blurred vision, difficulty passing urine, and loss of appetite.
Chloral drugs Chloral hydrate is one of the oldest sleeping drugs still in use	**chloral hydrate** *(Noctec, Welldorm)*	Chloral hydrate depresses brain function. It is generally considered to be less effective than benzodiazepines.	These drugs can quickly become ineffective, leading people to take greater and greater doses to achieve sleep.
Barbiturates Widely used until the 1960s, these drugs are no longer prescibed for sleeping problems because of the risks associated with overdose and addiction	**amylobarbitone** **butobarbitone** **quinalbarbitone**	These are central nervous system depressants that work by blocking the stimulatory chemical signals between nerve cells and the brain and reduce the ability of the cells to respond.	Side effects can include staggering, excessive sleepiness, and sometimes excitability. There is a high risk of respiratory depression. The effects of the drugs are greatly increased when combined with alcohol. Barbiturates are controlled drugs in most countries.

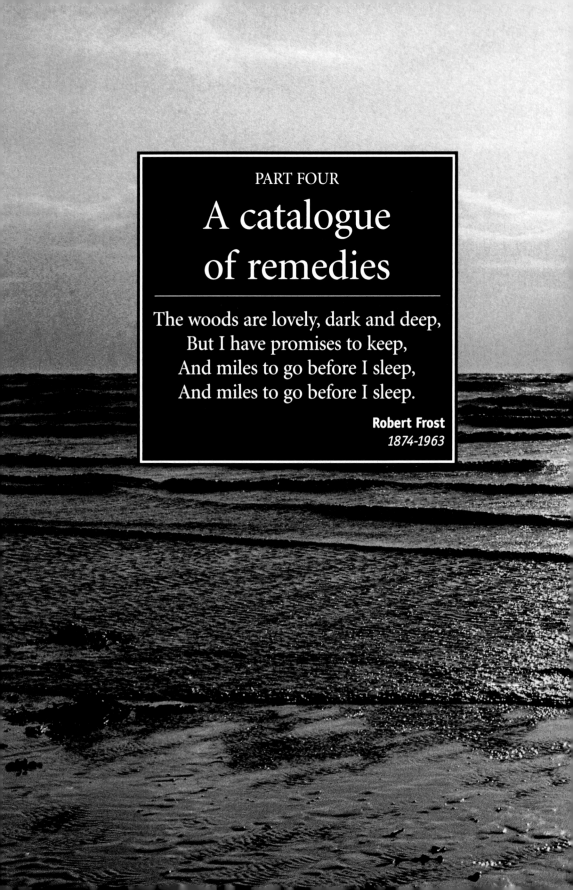

PART FOUR

A catalogue of remedies

The woods are lovely, dark and deep,
But I have promises to keep,
And miles to go before I sleep,
And miles to go before I sleep.

Robert Frost
1874-1963

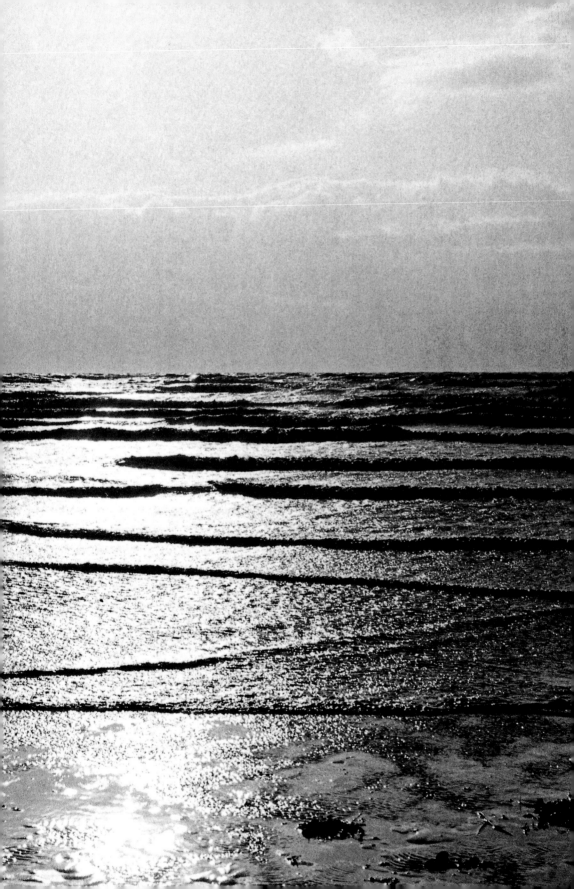

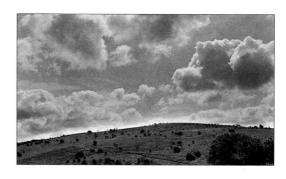

Selecting a natural remedy

There are many natural remedies for sleeplessness. Aromatherapy, herbalism, homeopathy, yoga, and relaxation techniques have all been shown to help with sleep disorders and improve health generally, with none of the side effects of sleeping pills. Using natural remedies, combined with improvements in lifestyle, may improve your sleep without the need for further help. However, if your sleeping problem has not resolved within a few weeks, you should seek expert help from an orthodox medical doctor or qualified complementary therapist.

How natural therapies can help

Complementary treatment for insomnia is not aimed simply at making you sleep better, but at restoring your mind, body, and emotions to a state of balance, which allows you to function more efficiently, heal more effectively and remain more in control of your waking and sleeping life. Sleep disorders tend to be resolved as a consequence of this restoration of balance rather than as a direct result of taking a sleep remedy.

Natural remedies do not provide miraculous cures. Some people do see an instant improvement in their sleep problems, for others it is a gradual process of recovery. No therapy can compensate for the adverse effects of bad diet, too many cigarettes, too much alcohol, too little exercise, and poor stress management. So rethink your lifestyle as well as trying to alleviate your immediate problem.

Seeking professional advice

Choose a complementary therapist with care. The vast majority of natural therapies are not state regulated, which means that anyone with the minimum of qualifications can set themselves up as a practitioner. Most therapies, however, are governed by self-regulating bodies, which ensure that their members work to a code of conduct, are insured to practise, and are subject to disciplinary procedures should they be found guilty of malpractice. If you want to find a complementary therapist contact one of the organizations listed on pp.156-7.

Using natural therapies safely

Complementary treatments are generally safe and can be very effective. However, certain precautions are sensible. Do not take remedies for longer than you need to, check the safety guidelines for use, especially for children, and keep all medicines out of the reach of children.

Choosing a therapy

All the remedies and exercises in this section are safe and easy to use at home. They are also effective, but not all remedies are effective for everyone and not every system of medicine suits everyone. Your best guide to choosing a therapy is to combine knowledge with intuition. Read through the descriptions of each therapeutic system and the lists of remedies and try the therapies to which you feel most attracted. Some people are drawn to the sensual fragrances of aromatherapy, others prefer to take a herbal preparation, or enjoy the ritual involved in making a herbal tea every night before bedtime. For others homeopathic remedies may seem to offer the simplest alternative. However, taking a homeopathic remedy requires a certain amount of self-knowledge. It is virtually impossible to be objective about oneself so, if you do not consult a homeopath, ask a friend to help you choose a remedy. A technique such as self-hypnosis will not suit everyone. Some people are fascinated by the power of the mind, others are frightened by it. It is not an instant solution; it takes practice and dedication to obtain results.

Many of the natural therapies can be used together. For example, you can safely combine a relaxing aromatherapy bath with a herbal sleep remedy without risk.

The natural remedies

A brief introduction to each of the listed therapies and remedies is provided in this section. While all of these complementary therapies have a wide range of applications in the maintenance of good health and the treatment of disease, the information here focuses on their use in the context of sleeping problems.

Yoga

This ancient system of exercise is suitable for people of all ages and levels of ability. Simple stretching and relaxation exercises modified to suit your health and level of fitness can increase suppleness, enhance mental and physical relaxation, and improve the quality of your sleep. The most important thing is to practise regularly. Doing these simple exercises every evening will help you to go to sleep free from tension and with a calm and relaxed mind.

Basic guidelines

♦ Check with your doctor before beginning any exercise regime, particularly if you are elderly, disabled, taking medication, epileptic, or suffer from any other chronic illness.
♦ Do not exercise on a full stomach.
♦ Choose a peaceful, warm, well-ventilated area. Wear clothes that allow you to stretch comfortably.
♦ Exercise in bare feet on a non-slip surface.
♦ Generally, breathe in as you move into a posture and breathe out as you stretch into the posture, unless otherwise instructed. Breathe slowly and deeply, making your "out" breath longer than your "in" breath.
♦ Make sure your lower back is comfortable and supported during any postures in which you are lying on the floor.

Best for
Yoga relaxation, which uses breathing and a visualization technique, is particularly suitable for the elderly and physically disabled who may be unable to undertake more vigorous forms of exercise.

Your three-step programme
The following programme of yoga exercises is organized as a three-part sequence designed to help you unwind mentally and physically and prepare for sleep.
Step one: Use breathing techniques to relax for five minutes to unwind from daily activities.
Step two: Do gentle stretches for ten minutes. When doing the exercises listen to your body and be guided by it. Stretch only as far and as often as is comfortable, and do only those postures you can achieve comfortably.
Step three: Use breathing relaxation or yoga nidra for ten minutes.

Breathing and unwinding

1 Lie on the floor as shown. Make sure that your lower back is comfortable.

2 Relax your face. Close your eyes and relax your tongue. Breathe in and out slowly and evenly through both nostrils.

3 Focus on the breath flowing gently into your abdomen. Feel the chest moving up and the ribcage expanding outward then the diaphragm moving downward and your abdomen rising. Exhale longer than you inhale.

4 Pause between each breath and repeat this abdominal breathing pattern until your mind feels calm and your body relaxed.

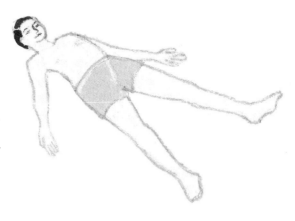

Stretches

Listen to your body throughout the session, keeping the mind focused on your stretch. Hold each stretch for a count of five to ten, depending on your flexibility. None of the postures should be painful, so stop you experience pain or discomfort at any time.

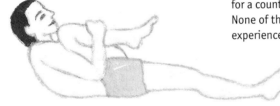

Leg stretches

1 Lying on your back bring your legs together and keep your arms by your sides. Inhale and at the same time bend your right leg in toward your chest and clasp your hands around the knee.

2 As you breathe out, bring your knee in to the chest. Repeat this twice.

3 Inhale and push your right leg straight up into the air with toes pointing toward the ceiling. Clasp the leg behind the knee or thigh to hold it straight. Gently stretch your heel up toward the ceiling.

4 Release your stretch slowly by counting to five and point your toes toward the ceiling. Bend your leg, lower and straighten it on the floor. Relax and repeat with the left leg, and then with both legs together.

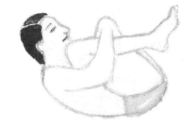

Lower back massage

1 Lying on your back with knees bent and feet flat on the floor, slightly lift your bottom and adjust your lower back so that it is in contact with the floor.

2 Inhale, bring your knees to your chest and clasp your hands around them. Gently rotate your knees clockwise several times. Repeat the rotations in an anti-clockwise direction. Rest your feet on the floor.

Supine spinal stretch

1 With both legs bent close to your chest, keeping thighs, knees, and feet together, breathe in and spread your arms out, with palms flat on the floor and fingers spread.

2 Exhale and bring both knees toward your right armpit. Turn your head to your left. Try to keep your left shoulder on the floor. Hold the stretch for three or four breaths.

3 Repeat the stretch on the other side. Place your feet on the floor with your legs bent.

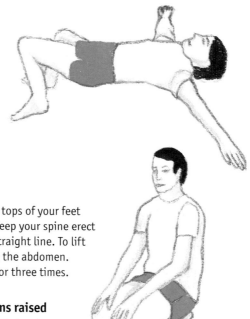

Sitting postures

Sit on your heels, keeping the tops of your feet flat on the floor, if possible. Keep your spine erect and your head and neck in a straight line. To lift your spine safely, pull up from the abdomen. Inhale and exhale deeply two or three times.

Side stretches – both arms raised

1 Sitting as above, place both hands beside your hips with fingertips touching the floor. Inhale and lift both hands together toward the ceiling, as shown.

2 Exhale and lean to the right, pressing the palms together. Inhale and return to the centre. Repeat for the left side.

Side stretches – one arm raised

1 Put your right hand on the floor, as shown. Spread your fingers and press your flat hand into the floor. Inhale and raise your left hand upward, lifting from the waist. Exhale and lean to the right. Hold for one or two breaths.

2 Inhale and return to the centre with a lift. Exhale and lower your hands to the floor. Repeat for the other side.

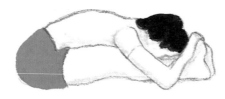

Back and hamstring stretch

1 Sitting upright with your legs together straight out in front, place your hands on your knees. Inhale and raise both hands over your head.

2 Exhale and bend forward to hold your feet, ankles, calves, or knees. Lower your head toward your knees. Inhale and come up slowly to an upright position.

Standing stretches

Stand with your legs hip width apart, feet parallel, and spine lifted up with head and neck in a straight line. Push your heels and toes into the floor. Inhale and exhale deeply a few times *(below left)*.

Gentle swings

Stand with feet slightly apart and knees slightly bent. Gently swing both arms first to the right, turning your head to the right. Then swing to the left, turning your head to the left. Repeat several times in a continuous movement. Relax with your legs together and arms by your sides.

Whole body stretch

Inhaling deeply, raise your arms above your head with hands clasped, and come up on to your toes. Stretch the whole body upward. Exhale and bring your arms to your side, and lower your heels to the floor. Repeat once more.

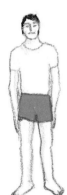
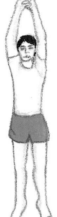
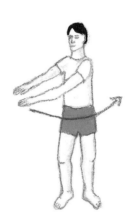

Yoga nidra relaxation

1 Lying in the same position as for Breathing and unwinding (p.137), breathe deeply and evenly through both nostrils for several seconds. Feel the in breath flow right down into your abdomen and as you exhale let any remaining tension in your body flow out with it.

2 Visualize a relaxing scene. Focus on your feet. Tense and release your toes, then flex your feet hard and as you relax them feel all the tension drain from your feet, ankles, calves, knees, thighs, buttocks, and abdomen and breathe it out.

3 Focus on your hands. Tense the muscles in your arms and hands by clenching your hands into a tight fist, release and let the tension flow from your fingertips up your arms to your shoulders. Breathe it out.

4 Focus on your shoulders. Tense your shoulder blades and relax them three times.

5 Turn your head to right and left to free any tension in the neck muscles and let your neck relax. Finally tense your facial muscles and as you release them be aware of all the tension draining out of the areas of tension, around your jaw and mouth, the eyes, and away from the forehead.

Self-hypnosis

The word "hypnosis" describes a trance-like state between waking and sleeping. When used in conjunction with improvements to sleep hygiene, hypnosis is an effective aid to improving the quality of your sleep. It is easiest to learn self-hypnosis from a therapist. However, it is also possible to teach yourself. Hypnosis is perfectly safe as you cannot be hypnotized unless you want it to happen. Nobody can make you do something under hypnosis that you would not normally do – your subconscious will reject any suggestion it deems unethical.

There are many ways to induce hypnosis. The technique described here is fairly typical. It is important to make sure that nothing disturbs you as you go through the self-hypnosis routine. It may take you some time to go into a hypnotic state when you are starting and it is not unusual for this to take 20 minutes or more at first. However, with practice it will happen much more rapidly. Do not be surprised if you do not feel as if you are in a trance. Hypnosis simply feels like a state of deep relaxation.

Cautions

Those who are mentally unstable or who have a history of psychiatric problems should seek professional advice before undertaking self-hypnosis. If you consult a hypnotherapist, make sure that he or she is registered with a recognized body and insured to practise.

Make your own sleep tape

It is impossible to go into hypnosis while reading instructions so it is a good idea to read the technique on to a tape in a slow, relaxed voice, and play it back to yourself when you go to bed. You can play some gentle atmospheric music as a background to your tape, if you find this relaxing. Alternatively, you can buy a self-hypnosis tape that comes complete with a guided visualization exercise.

Best for

Self-hypnosis works best for people who are ready and willing to change their habits and are prepared to practise the technique regularly.

How to induce self-hypnosis

1 Lie down with your legs slightly apart and your hands not touching. Take a deep breath and release it slowly. Be aware of any tension in your toes, clench them tight and release them, imagining them lengthening and relaxing. Work up through the muscles of your feet, calves, and thighs, tensing and releasing them so that they feel soft and heavy. Focus on your breathing, keeping it slow and regular, and tell yourself that every time you breathe out you will feel more and more relaxed.

2 Tense and release the muscles in the lower back and abdomen, in your chest, shoulders, and through the upper arms, forearms, hands, and fingers. Let tension flow out through your fingertips.

3 Tense and relax your neck muscles. Imagine the tension in your face being smoothed out by gentle fingertips. Then let the tension flow from your scalp.

4 Continue to breathe slowly and deeply. As you release each breath become aware of the last drops of tension gently trickling out of your body. Tell yourself that you have nothing to do but relax. Think only of the breath moving in and out of your body.

5 Without lifting your head, fix your eyes on a spot on the ceiling. Roll your eyes back as if you were looking for your eyebrows. Keeping your gaze fixed on the spot on the ceiling, take four long deep breaths. Inhale and hold for a count of ten, and as you exhale tell yourself to "sleep now". Repeat four times, holding your breath progressively longer.

6 Allow a floating sensation to flow through your body and picture ten steps in front of you. Look down the steps into a beautiful garden below. Try to see, smell, and sense the garden. Start to walk down the steps counting backward from ten to one with each step. As you step down each step, tell yourself that you feel more and more relaxed. Tell yourself that when you take the final step you will be deeply relaxed.

7 Next find a place in your garden where you would like to fall asleep. Tell yourself, "I am moving into deep and restful sleep." Focus on a positive image of yourself dozing peacefully. Lie still and relaxed and keep breathing steadily.

8 You may fall asleep during the exercise or soon afterward. If not, tell yourself, "On the count of one I will return to full awareness. On the count of two I will feel relaxed. On the count of three I will wake feeling relaxed and ready to enjoy restorative sleep." Then count to three, open your eyes, stretch, take a long deep breath, and settle down to sleep.

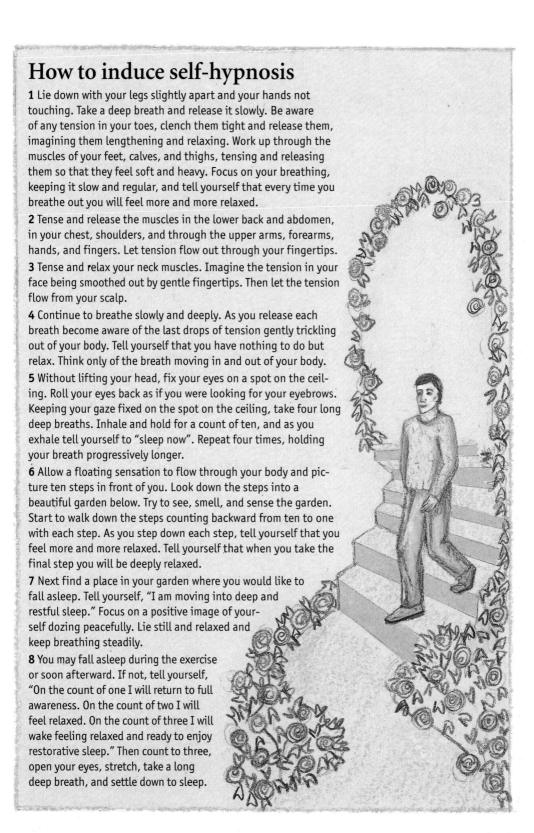

Homeopathic remedies

Homeopathy is based on the principle of treating like with like. A remedy is taken to match the symptoms of your disease in the belief that two similar diseases cannot exist in the body at the same time. Introducing a harmless copy-cat disease can drive out the harmful original before dying off itself.

The curative substance is diluted by a process known as succussion so that no detectable trace of it remains. The remedies do not work in any chemical way, but are said to hold a vibrational or energetic pattern of the original substance that stimulates an individual's natural healing abilities, or "vital force".

Professional homeopaths do not generally prescribe remedies to treat symptoms individually, as the symptoms are considered to be only the outward sign that your vital force is struggling to overcome disease. Instead a remedy is prescribed for the whole person. Accurate prescribing is essential to the success of homeopathy. Although your chances of obtaining the right remedy are obviously far greater if you consult a qualified homeo-path, self-prescribing can often work for minor problems. When choosing a homeopathic remedy you may be faced with six or seven possibilities; the skill in self-prescribing lies in being able to choose the correct remedy from those possibilities.

The table on pp.144-5 lists a range of types of sleeping problem and symptoms together with appropriate remedies. Choose 6c potency to be taken every half hour for acute problems or once daily for more established conditions. Continue treatment for two to three weeks. If there is no improvement within this time, stop taking the

Best for

People who know themselves pretty well or are interested in the detail involved in prescribing for the individual.

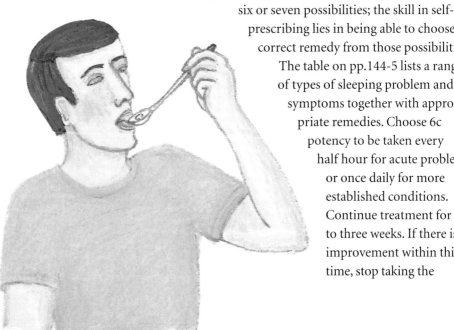

remedy and try a different one or consult a qualified homeopath for further advice.

Homeopathic remedies will not interfere with orthodox medical treatments, although some drugs may impair the benefits of homeopathic remedies. Strong smells also affect how well homeopathic remedies work. Some practitioners advise against using aromatherapy oils in conjunction with homeopathic remedies.

How to take the remedies

Homeopathic remedies are available from many pharmacies and healthfood stores, and from specialist suppliers. They come in the form of tiny lactose tablets, granules, powders, or liquid. The remedy should be taken in a "clean" mouth, meaning you should leave at least 30 minutes between taking the remedy and eating, drinking, cleaning the teeth, or smoking. Take only one remedy at a time and try not to touch the tablets. Empty a pill onto a teaspoon, tuck it under your tongue, and allow it to dissolve. Crush the tablet on to a spoon for babies. Store homeopathic remedies in a cool dark place, away from strong smells.

Using the homeopathic remedy finder

A remedy profile includes many aspects of the individual's health and physical constitution. Look for your key symptom(s) and list all the remedies that relate to those symptoms. Next look for the secondary symptoms and list in order of preference those remedies that match your symptoms and/or constitution. To narrow the selection even further work through the information in the "feels better" and "feels worse" columns.

One remedy may stand out as the right one for you, but it is possible that you might not be able to choose between two remedies. In this case take one of the remedies for a few days and if you do not start to sleep better, try your second choice.

Cautions

Homeopathic remedies are perfectly safe and can work wonderfully for babies, but as with all medicines, treat them responsibly and do not continue to take a remedy that is not working for you.

Homeopathic remedy finder

KEY SYMPTOMS	OTHER SYMPTOMS	FEELS BETTER	FEELS WORSE	REMEDY
Acute insomnia caused by shock, fright, bad news, or grief.	Fear, anxiety, and restlessness. May be woken by nightmares.	For fresh air, in a cool room.	At night, in a warm stuffy room, for cigarette smoke, heavy or stifling bedclothes.	Aconite
Waking between 1am-3am because of anxiety or an overactive mind.	Sleepy during the day but anxious at night. Restless in bed with anxious dreams and nightmares.	For warmth, warm drinks, moving about, and sleeping propped up in bed.	For being cold or alone, drinking alcohol.	Arsenicum album
Nightmares, waking around 3-4am feeling bright and cheerful, and not sleeping again until just before normal getting up time.	Sleeplessness due to irritability, overwork, or working late. Easily disturbed by light and noise. Drowsy in the evening and after food.	For warmth, in the evening, and when left alone.	For alcohol, overeating – especially spicy foods, noise, lack of sleep.	Nux vomica
Sleeplessness caused by shock, emotional stress, or grief.	Jerks limbs when falling asleep. Mood swings, no thirst, dreams with bottled up anger and tension.	For distractions.	For coffee and alcohol, for cold or fresh air. Craves, but worse for, sweets.	Ignatia
Night terrors, or waking with a sinking feeling in the stomach. Caused by excitement or mental strain.	Anxiety, irritability, and muscle fatigue. Exhausted by stress or overwork.	For warmth and gentle movement, after eating.	For exertion, excitement or worry, in winter, for cold, between 3-5am.	Kali phos
Early waking with an overactive mind and/or recurrent thoughts.	Anxious or vivid dreams, night sweats. Throws off bed clothes feeling too hot, but pulls them back because of cold.	In a cool room with fresh air, for gentle activity during the day, for cool drinks and affection.	During the evening, in a stuffy room, for cold or staying still.	Pulsatilla
Difficulty falling asleep. Waking early feeling unrefreshed. Exhausted and depressed by overwork and mental stress.	Feels irritable and sleepy during the day. Suffers headaches, nausea, and dizziness due to tiredness. Night sweats.	For naps, vigorous exercise, fresh air, and a warm bed.	For lack of physical activity, emotional stress, before a period, during a thunderstorm or heavy weather.	Sepia
Inability to relax due to the over-excitement caused by good news or ideas.	Vivid dreams, overactive mind, over-excitement.	For lying down in a warm room.	For cold or fresh air, sleeping pills, stimulants, noise, too much excitement.	Coffea

KEY SYMPTOMS	OTHER SYMPTOMS	FEELS BETTER	FEELS WORSE	REMEDY
Wetting the bed during dreams.	Nervous-system immaturity.	After a nap, lying on the back.	For movement, pressure or touch, and while lying on the right side.	**Equisetum**
Bedwetting in the early part of the night.	Over-sensitive child, easily upset and tearful. Afraid of the dark. Strong sense of justice.	In a warm bed.	In winter.	**Causticum**
Awakened by the slightest noise and finds it difficult to get back to sleep. Feels hot and thrusts limbs out from under the covers.	Kept awake by a continuous flow of ideas. Vivid nightmares, disturbed and unrefreshing sleep, waking in the early hours then sleeping late.	After short naps, for lying on the right side.	On waking in the morning and at night, in stuffy rooms or a hot bed. For stimulants.	**Sulphur**
Sleep problems during the menopause. Sensation of suffocation at the throat or bed swaying as you go to sleep.	Dread of going to bed because of sudden awakenings and the sensation of swaying. Tendency to hold breath while falling asleep. Night sweats. Waking anxious and feeling unwell.	For fresh air and when period starts.	In a warm or stuffy room, on waking up. For tight clothes.	**Lachesis**
Wakes up early and unrefreshed just before time to get up.	Pain where you have been lying, feeling cold, sleep-talking, anxious dreams, stress headaches.	For stretching and massage.	At night. For cold and damp, and for stimulants.	**Thuja**
Irritable baby who refuses to be calmed. Sleeplessness caused by teething, anger, or colic.	Moaning when asleep, eyes are half open when asleep.	In warm, damp weather, when carried or travelling in car.	After 9pm, after burping, in cold windy weather, when too hot.	**Chamomilla**
Difficulty waking and getting up in the morning, waking up before midnight. Painful teething in restless babies.	Anxious, irritable, sluggish, and restless. Dislikes routine. Babies who scream in their sleep and need lots of attention.	For cold, damp, draughts, fresh air, worry, grief or exertion.	In summer and in warm, dry weather.	**Calcerea phosphorica**

Herbal remedies

Herbalism involves using plants, flowers, trees, and herbs with healing properties to enhance our natural healing powers. Professional herbalists do not prescribe herbs simply to treat symptoms such as insomnia but aim to correct the imbalances within the body that cause those symptoms. For example, sedative herbs such as hops and valerian are used to relax the nervous system to that you enjoy natural, restorative sleep. Each herb contains a variety of active constituents and has a main action and several subsidiary actions which determine the conditions for which it is most appropriate.

There are numerous sleep-promoting herbs. You can buy these in a variety of over-the-counter preparations or obtain the individual dried herbs to make your own infusions and/or to use in your evening bath. To find an appropriate herb for your sleeping problem, consult a professional herbalist, who will base his or her recommendations on a full account of your history and symptoms. Alternatively, you can make your own selection from the table on pp.148-9.

Making a herb "tea"

To make a herbal infusion, use fresh or dried flowers, leaves, or the green stems of the plants. Add approximately 28g (1oz) of dried herbs to 600ml (1 pint) of boiling water. Cover and leave to infuse for 10 to 15 minutes. Then strain and drink hot.

With fresh herbs, use approximately a handful of the herb, making it stronger or weaker according to your taste. Sweeten the tea with honey if you prefer. Heat destroys the properties of valerian root, so it should be infused in cold water for up to 12 hours.

Decoctions are similar to infusions but the method is reserved for the hard, woody parts of plants. Using 28g (1oz) of herb to 750ml (1¼ pints) of water, put the herb and water in a saucepan and bring to the boil, simmer for 10 minutes, strain, and drink hot.

Reduce the dosage of herbs taken by mouth by a quarter for children under five years old and by a half for children under twelve.

How much and when

For insomnia take one or two cupfuls of an infusion or decoction in the evening about 30-60 minutes before bedtime. A further cup can be taken in the night if you wake up. Where a remedy that will not make you drowsy is indicated for conditions associated with insomnia you can take it three times a day.

Using the herbal remedy finder

Use the table on pp.148-9 to find the key herb most suited to your problem, taking into account any other symptoms you may have. You can take a herb on its own or combine it with another herb for additional benefits. Any herb that can be taken internally can also be used in the bath, either with other herbs or combined with essential oils.

Best for

Herbalism is most suitable for those who are prepared to take the remedies regularly and who do not expect instant results. Herbal remedies are particularly appropriate for people who enjoy the ceremony of preparing their evening infusion and have the time to do so.

External applications

Herbal baths are a pleasant way to use herbs for the alleviation of sleeping difficulties. The relaxing and warming effect of the hot water enhances the sedative properties of the herbs. Herbal baths can be used with herbal infusions. Add a litre (1¾ pints) of strained herbal infusion or decoction (left to brew for 30 minutes) to your bath water or tie a handful of herbs in a muslin bag and hang it from the hot-water tap so that the water runs through it.

The heat of the water releases the fragrance and activates the properties of the herbs, while opening the pores of your skin. The inhaled scent passes through the nervous system to the brain, while the properties absorbed through the skin pass into the bloodstream. The result is benefits for both mind and body.

Herbal remedy finder

HERB	PROPERTIES	GOOD FOR	HOW TO USE	CAUTIONS
Passion flower *Passiflora*	Calming and sleep inducing, relieves pain, and muscular spasms.	General insomnia, insomnia in asthmatics, hysteria, cramps, and nerve pain.	By mouth In bath	No known risks when taken as recommended.
Jamaica dogwood	Calming, eases pain and disturbing persistent thoughts.	Insomnia caused by nervous tension, pain, or menstrual pain.	By mouth In bath	This is a powerful remedy; do not exceed the recommended dosage.
Valerian *Valeriana officinalis*	Relaxing and sleep-inducing, relieves spasms, calms the digestion, and lowers blood pressure.	Severe insomnia and insomnia accompanied by pain, cramps, intestinal pain, wind, menstrual pain, tension, anxiety, and over-excitability.	By mouth In bath	Does not suit everyone. Can occasionally cause excitement. Do not exceed recommended dosage.
Hops *Humulus lupulus*	Relaxing, sleep-inducing, and antiseptic.	General insomnia, especially tension or anxiety-related, or associated with restlessness, indigestion or headaches.	By mouth In bath	Do not take if depressed. Do not take during the first three months of pregnancy.
Californian poppy	Sleep- inducing, relieves pain, and quietens disturbed feelings.	Menopausal insomnia, excitable and sleepless children, anxiety.	By mouth In bath	No known risks when taken as recommended.
Chamomile *Chamaemelum nobile*	Relaxing, eases digestion, relieves spasm, pain-relieving and antiseptic, helps to heal wounds.	Gentle remedy suitable for children. Good for anxiety, indigestion, inflammation, and catarrh.	By mouth In bath	No known risks when taken as recommended.
Balm	Calms the digestive system, lowers blood pressure, and relieves spasms.	Anxiety, depression, digestive spasms, stress.	By mouth In bath	No known risks when taken as recommended.
Oats	Excellent nerve tonic, antidepressant, nourishing.	Stress, exhaustion, depression, general illness or weakness, jet lag. Tranquillizer or sleeping pill withdrawal.	By mouth (as porridge) In bath	No known risks when taken as recommended.

HERB	PROPERTIES	GOOD FOR	HOW TO USE	CAUTIONS
St John's wort *Hypericum perforatum*	Sedative, pain-relieving, improves sleep quality.	Depression, anxiety, tension, insomnia, and hypersomnia, emotional upset during the menopause.	By mouth In bath	Prolonged use may increase sensitivity to sunlight.
Wild lettuce	Relaxing and sleep-inducing, relieves pain and destructive feelings.	Insomnia with rest-lessness and excitability. Good for overactive children, relieves muscular pains, painful periods, digestive cramps, and irritating coughs.	By mouth In bath	No known risks when taken as recommended.
Skullcap	Relaxing, nerve tonic, relieves spasms.	Insomnia with nervous tension, pre-menstrual syndrome, exhaustion, depres-sion, hysteria, stress.	By mouth In bat	No known risks when taken as recommended.

Cautions

Used correctly, herbal remedies are generally safe. But do not take any remedy unnecessarily, in greater doses or for longer than you need. Pregnant women, parents of babies requiring treatment, and those with a medical condition are advised to consult a qualified herbalist before taking any remedies. If you want to take herbal medicines in conjunction with conventional medicine, speak to both your family doctor and a herbalist.

Flower remedies

Flower essences are gentle remedies that are said to contain the "energy" or energetic imprint of a particular plant. The remedies are believed to work at a vibrational level within the body. The vibrations of our energy patterns can become imbalanced by stress, and emotional, dietary, and environmental factors. These imbalances can lead to symptoms such as headaches, indigestion, muscle tension, snoring, and insomnia. Each flower remedy is believed to vibrate at a particular frequency, and this property can be used to correct imbalances in our own energy systems. There are hundreds of flower essences from Europe, the Americas, Australia, and Asia. The flower remedies discovered by Dr Edward Bach over 60 years ago are perhaps the most famous of these.

Best for

Flower essences are useful for treating many types of sleeping problem, but are especially good for those of psychological or spiritual origin. They are extremely gentle and suitable for all ages. They do not interfere with other forms of treatment.

How to take a flower remedy

Flower remedies can be taken anywhere at any time. They require no preparation, have a pleasant taste, and have no dangerous side-effects. Take the remedy by dropping four drops onto your tongue at least four times a day or when you feel you need them. Alternatively, you can take the remedy in still spring water.

Using the flower essence remedy finder

To find a remedy appropriate for you, first check the "Suitable for" column. Look for a match for your problem or personality type and read across to find the recommended remedy. All the remedies are safe for general use.

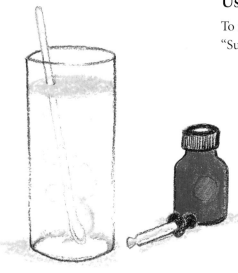

Many remedies are made by a number of manufacturers and are widely available. Others are exclusive to a particular manufacturer and may be less easy to find. Some manufacturers market combination remedies specifically for sleep problems. These are not listed here. Do not confuse flower remedies with aromatherapy oils or herbal preparations of the same name.

Flower essence remedy finder

REMEDY	SUITABLE FOR
Aspen	For those whose vague and irrational fears lead to night sweats, sleep-walking, and sleep-talking.
Banksia robur	For dynamic individuals who feel temporarily drained because of jet lag.
Black-eyed Susan	Impatient types who are always rushing and striving for success. Also for those who resist change and internal reflection, or repress disturbing memories and emotions.
Boronia	For those who are grieving, broken-hearted, or unable to sleep because of obsessive thoughts.
Chamomile	For people who are moody, easily angered or excited, and have difficulty calming down. Good for hyperactive children and for people with stress-sensitive digestive systems.
Dill	Good for jet lag and in times of stress or excessive stimulation. Also good for jetlagged children.
Green spider orchid	For nightmares and night terrors.
Lettuce	For those who are restless, excitable, and unable to concentrate.
Morning glory	For those with erratic sleep habits who find it difficult to get up in the morning and for those whose sleep is disturbed by stimulants and addiction to sleeping pills.
Rock rose	For nightmares brought on by a shock or accident.
Stock	For tense, nervous hyperative types dependent on stimulants, and prone to exhaustion and mood swings.
Valerian	For those who are restless at night and kept awake by pain or stress. Also for those who are exhausted or recovering from illness.
Verbena	For wound-up and hyperactive individuals. Use only before bedtime.
Vervain	For tense people who are unable to sleep owing to excitability.
Walnut	For those who find it hard to accept that we need less sleep as we age.
White chestnut	For people who cannot switch off to their mental chatter and are tormented by recurring thoughts of arguments or conversations they have had throughout the day.
Ylang ylang	Good for jet lag and for insomnia caused by stress or emotional upheaval.

Aromatherapy

Aromatherapy is the name given to the therapeutic use of essential oils. These are the distilled aromatic extracts of plants and flowers. Essential oils are easily inhaled or absorbed through the skin. Once in the body, they are carried in the bloodstream to the brain and body systems, where they exert their healing benefits on mind and body. All stress-related conditions, including insomnia, respond well to aromatherapy. Two or three oils can be blended together to combine their properties. Do not use undiluted oils on the skin and do not take them internally.

How to use essential oils

Massage is probably the most effective way of using essential oils. The combination of soothing touch and the therapeutic benefits of essential oils relaxes physical and mental tension. The drawback is that you need someone to massage you, so if you have not got a willing and able partner, you will need to consult an aromatherapist for treatment. The benefits last for hours so even if you have your massage in the afternoon it will still help you sleep.

For skin application the essential oil must be diluted in a vegetable carrier oil such as cold-pressed sunflower oil or sweet almond oil. Use 7-10 drops of essential oil to 25ml (five teaspoons) of carrier oil for adults, half that strength for children under seven and half again for children under the age of three. It is best not to use essential oils on newborn babies.

Any oil can be used in the bath, add 5-10 drops for adults, half that for children over two, and only one drop of a very gentle oil such as chamomile or lavender for younger children. Inhalation is also effective. Put one or two drops of a relaxing oil onto a handkerchief and tuck it inside your pillow to help you sleep.

Using the aromatherapy remedy finder

Check the "Properties" and "Uses" columns to find the essential oil that fits your case most closely.

Best for

Most people can benefit from aromatherapy. Take extra care with babies or very young children and if you are pregnant. If you do have an allergy or a chronic medical condition such as eczema, epilepsy, or high blood pressure, consult a qualified practitioner for treatment.

Aromatherapy remedy finder

ESSENTIAL OIL	PROPERTIES	USES	CAUTIONS
Benzoin *Styrax benzoin*	Sedative, warming, and relaxing.	Sleeplessness caused by worry, emotional exhaustion, tension, bronchitis, and coughs.	Some people may be sensitive to this oil.
Clary sage *Salvia sclarea*	Warming and relaxing, antidepressant, lowers blood pressure, calms nervous system, aphrodisiac.	Depression, headache, stress, digestive cramps, asthma, high blood pressure, menopause.	Do not combine with alcohol.
German and Roman chamomile *Matricaria chamomilla and Chamaemele nobile*	Calms nerves and stomach, sleep inducing, especially good for children.	Insomnia, anxiety.	Can cause dermatitis in some people.
Jasmine *Jasminum officinalis*	Relaxing and soothing, antidepressant, sedative, aphrodisiac, expectorant.	Insomnia, depression, apathy, nervous exhaustion, stress, catarrh, breathing difficulties.	Non-toxic, non-irritant.
Lavender *Lavendula officinalis*	Calming, soothing to nerves and digestion, antidepressant, pain-relieving, lowers blood pressure.	Insomnia, tension, depression, headache, catarrh, stomach cramps, shock, earache.	Non-toxic, non-irritant.
Melissa *Lemon balm, Melissa officinalis*	Relaxing and uplifting, lowers blood pressure, helps digestion, menstruation, and nervous system.	Insomnia, nervous tension, depression, high blood pressure, indigestion, coughs, colds, shock, anxiety.	Use small amounts only as skin irritation is possible.
Neroli *Citrus aurantium amara*	Very relaxing.	Insomnia caused by anxiety, depression, irritability, panic, shock.	Non-toxic, non-irritant.
Rose *Rosa damascena*	Relaxing and soothing, aphrodisiac, nervous and digestive tonic, helps menstruation.	Insomnia, nervous tension, depression, headaches, painful periods, nausea, asthma, loss of sex drive.	Non-toxic, non-irritant.
Sandalwood *Santalum album*	Relaxing, aphrodisiac and antidepressant, expectorant, calms digestion.	Insomnia, depression, nervous tension, catarrh, colic.	Non-toxic, non-irritant.
Sweet marjoram *Origanum marjorana*	Warming and comforting, sedative, aids digestion and nervous functions.	Insomnia, anxiety, colds, catarrh, intestinal spasms, muscular and joint pain, headaches.	Non-toxic, non-irritant.
Ylang ylang *Cananga odorata genuina*	Relaxing, aphrodisiac, antidepressant, tones the nervous system, lowers blood pressure.	Insomnia, depression, stress, nervous tension, excitability.	Non-toxic, non-irritant.

Reflexology

Reflexology is a type of therapeutic foot massage. It is used to alleviate and prevent many types of illness, including stress-related conditions and problems relating to congestion. Reflexologists believe that every part of the body is reflected in reflex areas on the hands and feet. The head and neck, for example, are reflected in the toes, the pelvis is reflected in the heels, and the reflex areas of the spine follow the inside arch of each foot. Practitioners also believe that the body is divided into ten vertical zones or channels of energy, which run from the head down through the body and surface at the reflex areas on the hands and feet. All the body parts within a zone are linked by the same energy.

Best for

Anyone can use reflexology, but it is best suited to those people who find touch relaxing and particularly enjoy having their feet touched. If you do not like having your feet touched or have a fungal or infectious skin condition that makes them unsuitable for treatment, you can work on your hands instead.

Reflex areas used to promote sleep

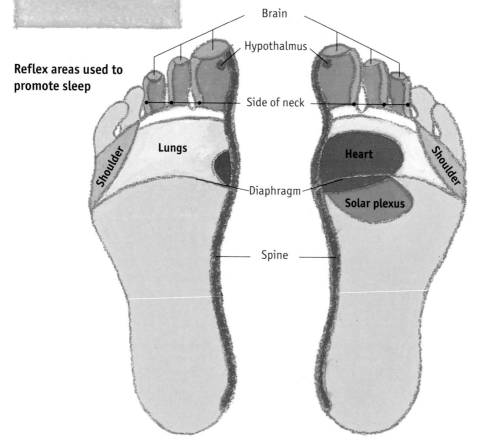

Brain

Hypothalmus

Side of neck

Shoulder

Lungs

Heart

Shoulder

Diaphragm

Solar plexus

Spine

By applying finger and thumb pressure to a specific point on the foot the therapist can stimulate or rebalance the energy in the related zone and improve the health of the associated body parts. Treatments are aimed at stimulating the body's own healing potential and are not given to "cure" any condition. Reflexology combines well with other complementary therapies.

Reflexology for restful sleep

Foot massage can be extremely soothing, whether you do it to yourself and especially if you have someone do it to you. Gently stroking the feet of a fractious baby can help to calm him or her down. Start every treatment by gently massaging the feet. When working the reflex areas keep your movements slow and rhythmic. Work over an area several times and when pressing into a point, hold for about 30 seconds. Give special emphasis to specific reflex points for insomnia, which include the reflexes for the brain, solar plexus, spine, respiratory, and circulatory systems (*see* facing page).

Cautions
Self-treatment is not advisable for pregnant women, diabetics, epileptics, or anyone receiving medical treatment. Use only very gentle stroking when treating babies and young children.

Self-administered reflexolgy
♦ Sit comfortably resting one bare foot on the other leg. Support your foot with your left hand (your right hand if left-handed) and work on the reflex points with your other hand.
♦ Begin by working all over the foot and then pay particular attention to the brain area at the top of your big toe and also on the top of your next two toes.
♦ Work your thumb from the middle of your big toe on the sole of your foot, up to the top of your toe. Repeat two or three times on each foot.
♦ Take a deep breath as you apply pressure to the solar plexus reflex point just below the ball of your foot. Exhale as you release the pressure. Repeat this three or four times to feel relaxed and sleepy.
♦ Thumb walk down the spinal reflexes on the inside arch of your foot to relieve spinal tension, pain, and stiffness. Work along the length of the spinal reflexes two or three times on each foot.
♦ To relax the respiratory system work up the sole of the foot from the base of the diaphragm line to the base of the toes. Using your index finger, work down the top of the foot from the grooves between the toes to the base of the lung area. Repeat on the other foot. Working this area also treats the heart reflexes that control circulation. Do not work excessively on this area.
♦ Finish by gently stroking all over the top of your feet from the toes down to the ankles on both feet.

Useful addresses

ACUPUNCTURE

The National Acupuncture
Foundation
1718 M Street, Suite 195
Washington, DC, 20036
Tel: (202) 332-5194
Provides information on accredited schools and practitioners.

AROMATHERAPY

Ayurvedic Foundations
Dean Campbell, President
P.O. Box 900413
Sandy, Utah 84090-0413
Tel: (801) 943-1480
Conducts workshops and custom training, produces audio cassette tapes, and provides Ayurvedic lifestyle counseling.

BIODYNAMIC MASSAGE

Contact the UK Council for
Psychotherapy (UKCP) or
The Gerda Boyesen Centre
Acacia House, Centre Avenue
London W3 7JX, UK
Tel: (44) 181-743-2437

CHINESE HERBALISM

Moonrise Herbs-EG
826 G Street
Arcata, California 95521
Tel: 1-800-603-8364
Fax: (707) 822-0506

Garden Supplements Symmetry
Independent Symmetry
Distributor
P.O. Box 831

Maywood, New Jersey 07607
Tel: 1-800-439-0381
Supplies entire botanical product line.

COLOR THERAPY

The International Association
for Color Therapy (IACT)
P.O. Box 3688
London SW13 0NX, UK
Tel: (44) 181-878-5276

FENG SHUI

Feng Shui Institute of America
P.O. Box 488
Wabasso, Florida 32970
Tel: (561) 589-9900
Fax: (561) 589-1611
website: http://www.windwater.com/.
Along with general information on Feng Shui, the Institute provides information on getting building plans approved by Feng Shui masters.

FLOWER THERAPY

The International Federation
for Vibrational Medicine
Middle Piccadilly Natural
Healing Centre, Holwell
Dorset, DT9 5LW, UK
Tel: (44) 1963-23468

The Edward Bach Centre
Mount Vernon
Sotwell, Wallingford
Oxon, OX10 0PZ, UK
Tel: (44) 1491-834678

HERBALISM

The National Institute of
Medical Herbalists
56 Longbrooke Street
Exeter EX4 8HA, UK
Tel: (44) 1392-426022
Further information about specific herbs can be found on the *website*: http://www.herbweb.com/.

HOMEOPATHY

The National Center for
Homeopathy
801 North Fairfax Street
Suite 306
Alexandria, Virginia 22314
Tel: (703) 548-7790
website: homeopathy@lyghtforce.com
provides a directory of licensed homeopathic practitioners

The American Association of
Naturopathic Physicians
2366 Eastlake Avenue
Suite 322
Seattle, Washington 98102
Tel: (206) 328-8510

KINESIOLOGY

The Siskiyou Essence Company
P.O. Box 563
Silver City
New Mexico 88062
Tel: (505) 388-0696
website: http://www.zianet.com/siskiyou.

REFLEXOLOGY

La Roche International College
Department Int1
P.O. Box 37, Scarborough, UK
Tel: (44) 1723-378573
website:
http://www.yorkshirenet.co.uk/businfo/lric/.

TAI CHI

Tai Chi Arts Association
212A Adams Street
Newton, Massachusetts 02158
Tel: (617) 969-1911
website: http://www.taichi-arts.com/.

YOGA

Yoga Institute of Washington
P.O. Box 27704
Washington, DC 20038
Tel: (301) 270-2111
website: http://www.yoga-institute.org/.

ORTHODOX MEDICAL PRACTITIONERS

American Sleep Apnea Assoc.
2025 Pennsylvania Avenue NW
Suite 905
Washington, DC 20006
Tel: (202) 293-3650
Fax: (202) 293-3656

Horizon Sleep Diagnostic
Centers
7850 Brookhollow Road
Dallas, Texas 75235
Tel: (214) 638-4352
Fax: (214) 638-4426
website: http://www.hsdcdal.com/info.htm.

Northside Hospital and Sleep
Disorders Center and Atlanta
School of Sleep Medicine and
Technology
1000 Johnson Ferry Road
Atlanta, Georgia 30342
Tel: (404) 851-8135

Sleep Disorders Institute
(Division of St. Luke's-
Roosevelt Hospital Center)
1090 Amsterdam Avenue
New York, New York 10025
Tel: (212) 523-1700

Stanford University Sleep
Disorders Center
701 Welch Road,
Suite 2226, Palo Alto
California 94304
Tel: (415) 725-6517
Fax: (415) 725-4913

Further Reading

JOURNALS

Contemporary Psychology
Journal of Behavioral Therapy
Psychology and Aging
Psychophysiology
Psychosomatic Medicine
Science
Sleep

BOOKS

Aromatherapy, an A-Z., Patricia
Davis (CW Daniel)
*The Audio Guide to Natural
Sleep*, P. Goldberg and D.
Kaufman (St. Martin's Press)
The Book of Ayurveda, Judith
Morrison (Fireside)

Dr. Spock's Baby and Child Care,
Dr. Benjamin Spock & Dr.
Michael Rothenberg (Dutton)
The Feng Shui Handbook, Master
Lam Kam Chuen (Henry Holt)
How to Get a Great Night's Sleep,
H. £ Pamela Vafi (Adams Pub.)
*The Illustrated Encyclopedia of
Essential Oils*, Julia Lawless
(Element)
*The Mammoth Dictionary of
Symbols*, Nadia Julien (Carroll &
Graf)
Natural Childhood, John
Thomson (Fireside)
The Natural House Book, David
Pearson (Fireside)
Restful Sleep, Deepak Chopra

(Harmony Books)
The Practice of Chinese Medicine,
Giovanni MacIoca (Churchill
Livingstone)
The Secret Language of Dreams,
David Fontana (Chronicle)
Secrets of Sleep, Alexander
Borbely (Basic Books)
The Sleep Book for Tired Parents,
R. Huntley (Parenting Press)
Sleep and Dreaming, Jacob
Empson (Harvester Wheatsheaf)
Sleep Without Drugs, Dr. Moses
Wong (Seven Hills Books)
*Understanding Dreams: How to
Benefit from the Power of Your
Dreams*, Nerys Dee
(HarperCollins)

Index

Acknowledgments

The author would like to thank all at Gaia, especially Cathy Meeus for all her hard work, guidance and patience; Dr Jacob Empson, Ronald C Chisholm PhD, for their expertise and advice; Margaret Ahmed of Sleep Matters and Greg Mader of the American Sleep Disorders Association for supplying valuable information; Pippa Duncan for her help with Part Three; yoga teacher Seema Khajuria for devising the yoga sequence in Part Four. Last but not least to Mick for his constant love and support.

Gaia Books would like to thank the following for their help in the preparation of this book: Lynn Bresler (proofreader), Jill Ford (indexer), Anne McIntyre, Gabriel Moje, Dr Helen Dziemidko, Anthony Porter, Dr Helen Engleman, and Jan Dunkley.

US Editor: Janice Easton

BESTSELLING BOOKS FOR THE HEALTH OF BODY AND MIND
THE GAIA SERIES - FROM FIRESIDE BOOKS

ACUPRESSURE FOR COMMON AILMENTS
by Chris Jarney and John Tindall
A step-by-step, instructional guide
that demystifies this ancient healing
art, teaching readers techniques to
treat over 40 chronic and acute ailments.
0-671-73135-1, $11.95

AROMATHERAPY FOR COMMON AILMENTS
by Shirley Price
This first-of-its-kind guide shows you
how to apply 30 of the most versatile
essential oils to treat more than 40
common health problems.
0-671-73134-3, $11.95

THE BOOK OF MASSAGE
by Lucy Lidell
From massage to shiatsu and reflexology, this book teaches you the
power of the human touch.
0-671-54139-0, $14.00

THE BOOK OF SHIATSU
by Paul Lundberg
The first detailed, step-by-step guide to
shiatsu–the ancient Oriental system of healing using hand pressure and gentle manipu-
lation to enhance health and well–being.
0-671-74488-7, $14.95

THE BOOK OF SOUND THERAPY
by Olivea Dewhurst-Maddock
Drawing on ancient wisdom and
modern science, this comprehensive
guide provides a practical introduction to using the power of music and
sound to cure, comfort, and inspire.
0-671-78639-3, $14.00

THE BOOK OF STRESS SURVIVAL
by Alex Kirsta
Learn to relax and stress-proof
your life-style with this comprehensive ref-
erence on stress and management.
0-671-63026-1, $14.00

HEALING WITH COLOR AND LIGHT
by Theo Gimbel
A practical guide that draws on both
ancient wisdom and modern science
to help you improve your mental,
physical, and spiritual health using
the potent energy of color and light.
0-671-86857-8, $14.00

HERBS FOR COMMON AILMENTS
by Anne McIntyre
This fully illustrated, self-help guide
presents safe and practical alternatives to orthodox medical practices,
providing step-by-step instructions
for preparing herbal remedies to treat
more than 100 common health problems.
0-671-74632-4, $12.00

NATURAL CHILDHOOD
General Editor, John Thompson
The first practical and holistic guide for
parents of the developing child.
0-02-020739-5, $20.00

THE NATURAL GARDEN BOOK
by Peter Harper
Stressing a holistic and organic
approach, this beautifully designed
book offers practical advice for creating an environmentally safe, self-
regulating garden–in any setting.
0-671-74487-9, $35.00, cloth
0-671-74323-6, $25.00, paper

THE NATURAL HOUSE BOOK
by David Pearson
foreword by Malcolm Wells
Combining home design with health
and environmental concerns, this
lavishly illustrated, comprehensive
handbook shows you how to turn
any house or apartment into a sanc-
tuary for enhancing your well-being.
0-671-66635-5, $20.00

THE SIVANANDA COMPANION TO YOGA
by The Sivananda Yoga Center
This classic guide to yoga offers
clear, easy-to-follow exercises covering all aspects of this timeless discipline, including physical postures,
breathing exercises, diet, relaxation
and meditation techniques.
0-671-47088-4, $14.00

STEP-BY-STEP TAI CHI
The Natural Way to Strength and Health
by Master Lam Kam Chuen
This easy-to-use manual explains the
system of exercise that's sweeping
the country–a highly effective form
of body work that requires little time
and minimum space.
0-671-89247-9, $14.00

THE TAO OF SEXUAL MASSAGE
by Stephen Russell and Jürgen Kolb
A step-by-step guide to the ancient
Taoist system of sexual massage that
will help you free your deepest and
most joyful sensual energies.
0-671-78089-1, $15.00

THE WAY OF ENERGY
by Master Lam Kam Cheun
The first step-by-step guide to this unique
and highly praised form of ancient Chinese
medicine–motionless exercises that
cleanse and strengthen your body and
actually generate energy.
0-671-73645-0, $14.95

YOGA FOR COMMON AILMENTS
**by Dr. Robin Monro, Dr. Nagarathna,
and Dr. Nagendra**
From cancer to the common
cold–this holistic guide shows you
how to use yoga to reduce inner tensions and heal the body naturally.
0-671-70528-8, $10.95